Through the Eyes

of a

Young Physician Assistant

Through the Eyes

of a

Young Physician Assistant

SEAN CONROY, PA-C

Open Books Press
Bloomington, Indiana

Published by Open Books Press, USA

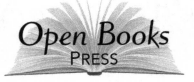

www.OpenBooksPress.com
info@OpenBooksPress.com

An imprint of Pen & Publish, Inc.
www.PenandPublish.com
Bloomington, Indiana
(314) 827-6567

Print ISBN: **978-1-941799-27-7**
eBook ISBN: **978-1-941799-28-4**

Library of Congress Control Number: **2016933348**

Printed on acid-free paper.

Cover Photo: Sean Conroy
Author Photo: Jessa Kennedy
Cover Design: Jennifer Geist

This book is dedicated to Briella Faith Quaduor, the angel who left too soon.

I would have never finished writing it without the love and support of my wife Shannon; my greatest supporter. A great deal of thanks is also due to Finley, Colin, Drew, Stephen, Sharon, Rod, and Deb for their support. Finally, I majored in medicine, not English, so this book was greatly enhanced by Vanessa Del Fabbro, and Jennifer Geist, who offered their editorial prowess.

Table of Contents

Introduction

This book was born out of my care of one particular patient during my Internal Medicine rotation in Grand Island, Nebraska: a gentleman facing his mortality. I had taken many small steps from lowly physician assistant student toward full-grown physician assistant. This patient was my first large step. In training in medicine there are many moments that affect you. These are the moments when, if you turn and look back on your education, you realize that you will never be the same again. Something inside me changed after my time with this gentleman. He was not my first patient to die, as you will quickly learn in the pages of this book. But he was the first "young" person that I lost. Sure, he had a granddaughter, but he was young to be a grandfather, and he was too young to die. It was after caring for him that a spark inside me grew into a burning desire to share his story and the stories of others, not only because his story moved me so much, but because I felt his story would move others if I found a way to share it.

I have read numerous books by physicians looking back on their formative years. Every good preceptor will ask if you have read *The House of God* by Samuel Shem. I have, but it was written in the seventies, and medicine has grown so much since then. Furthermore, though excellent, it is a work of fiction. It was like a gateway drug into medical literature. After reading it, I launched into *First Do No Harm* (Lisa Belkin), *Intern Blues* (Robert Marion), *Complications* and *Better* (Atul Gawande), and *Final Exam* (Pauline W. Chen)—all marvelous books and all worth reading, yet all written by physicians. I looked around but did not find any books by physician assistants that were not study guides, ethics books, histories of the profession, or specialty-specific books, such as cardiology, pediatrics, etc. I saw an area of literature not yet served: a first-person perspective on the early molding of PAs.

Having mentioned the books that served as inspiration to write this book, I fear paling in comparison. It was only with great prodding by my wife that, after beginning this book and losing steam for two years, I dove back in, finished it, and submitted it for publication. She read the first, and roughest, draft and pushed me to finish and publish it. Despite her faith in me, I don't know if I can match the authors I have mentioned, but my book can at least tell the stories I find so moving and keep those who live in my memory alive just a bit longer as their stories are transferred to paper. Perhaps my book will serve as inspiration for those who are uncertain of their career path and lead them to become physician assistants as well. Perhaps they, too, will be touched by patients' stories that beg to be told, and someday their books will sit side-by-side with mine on bookshelves. In the end, I wrote this book for myself: to share the stories of patients that affected me deeply and made me who I am. And, in doing so, others can now observe the world of medicine from a vantage point not yet shown: through the eyes of a young PA.

Family Practice I
Chadron, Nebraska

In June 2009, after surviving the didactic, or classroom-based phase of my training as a physician assistant, it was time for me to take the book knowledge and limited skills I had developed while "examining" my classmates and launch into the clinical field of study with real patients. My school wisely started each PA student on an easier rotation—family practice, general surgery, pediatrics, etc.—to gently acclimate us to the real world of medicine. I opted for family practice in Chadron, the small Nebraska town where I had been an undergraduate student at Chadron State College. All of my rotations were completed in the state of Nebraska—my own doing—because I chose not to venture too far from my wife and two sons, although others in my class set up rotations across the country. With little time between rotations and travel up to me to schedule, it was easier to keep them all within driving distance of school. This first rotation, interestingly enough, took me farther from my home in Lincoln, Nebraska than any other. My best friend from high school and college roommate, Alex, had agreed to let me stay with him so I wouldn't have to live in the call room at the hospital for four weeks. The hospitals my school used provided room and board, but I wanted the chance to reconnect with an old friend—and avoid eating out of the hospital cafeteria the whole time. The worst part about having to travel for rotations was carrying a milk crate of my books from my car to my room. This milk crate weighed between thirty and forty pounds. I would come to learn that even though I could park close to my dorm at most of my rotations, the room for the student was usually at the end of a very long hallway. I soon learned that I didn't need *all* of my books for each rotation. Alex was taking pictures for our alma mater at the annual golf tournament when I arrived in town. We met up, I got the key to his house, and quickly settled into his basement with my milk crate of books.

Although I spent the weekend relaxing with my best friend at his house, on Monday morning I was still one nervous little PA student as I walked into the hospital on the first day of my first rotation. I was told to look for my preceptor at the nurses' station, of which there was only one in this small Nebraska hospital. Janet the PA greeted me and said we would soon be departing for the Job Corps twelve miles south of town. Upon our arrival, Janet assigned me the one menial task a rookie was expected to handle: an H and P or a history and physical exam. I had to go see the patient, assess what problems I thought they had, and create a treatment plan. Then I had to present this patient (in ninety seconds or less) to my preceptor (in this case Janet), so that she could make the final decision. This is the education model followed by virtually every medical program in the world with experienced medical professionals acting as preceptors to residents, PA/Nurse Practitioner students, and sometimes even first-year medical students.

On this first rotation I did not see a single patient on my own; there was always a qualified provider following me, watching diligently. When I was on emergency department, ED, call there were mostly sports injuries and a few cuts needing sutures. For the most part, there were no grave emergencies. There were no patients that I felt I could not handle, especially with my preceptor watching so closely. I could almost feel her breathing down my neck at times. In the clinic, there were mostly annual physical exams, late-arriving summertime colds, and sprained ankles for me to diagnose and treat. The best part about clinical rotations was that I was encouraged to investigate disease and interesting cases on my own. Most of my knowledge was gained during the day discussing patients with my preceptors without the dread of an imminent test, which would only be administered once a quarter when my classmates and I returned to campus for meetings. This left time—barring a patient in the emergency department—for Alex and me to catch up and hang out in the evenings after clinic hours. I had brought all of my notes from lectures during the first two years of school and would review them while we watched the NBA playoffs, which were winding down during my stay in Chadron.

As with the ED and clinic, there was not much excitement on the hospital side either. I only had one person to perform daily rounds on my entire stay in Chadron: an elderly female admitted to the floor from the ED after a severe flare-up of her previously diagnosed diverticulitis[1]. Estelle presented to the ED one Saturday afternoon with left lower-quadrant pain, nausea, and a low-grade fever. She was visibly anxious and expressed fear she had brought this on herself because she had eaten Corn Nuts the night before. For people with diverticulitis, foods that can become lodged in a diverticulum are off limits. These include popcorn due to un-popped kernels, seeds, corn, and nuts. For

---

1   A condition where small pouches form in the colon, most common in the left lower abdominal area

this reason certainly Corn Nuts would be off limits for Estelle. In fact, when I first met her she was cussing herself up one side and down the other. I did my best to alleviate her fears and began a grueling abdominal exam. Anything that inflames the lining of the abdominal cavity causes a great deal of pain. The only way to localize and assess this pain, unfortunately, is to press on the abdomen until the pain is found, or to press on an area close by and allow the abdomen to snap back upward, stretching the inflamed lining. It did not take long to tell that she most likely did have an inflammation of this lining, since every gentle touch, prod, and movement elicited a moan. The test of choice—the one I recommended and my preceptor ordered—was a CT scan to see if she had ruptured a diverticulum. If this indeed were the case, she would have to be dealt with quickly, because she would then be suffering from an inflammation of the abdominal cavity known as peritonitis. Since it was the weekend, the radiology tech would have to be called in, and the test would take an extensive amount of time. My preceptor told me to go home and that she would call me if the CT showed a ruptured diverticulum. I asked if I would be allowed to scrub in for the emergency surgery if it were required. She didn't see why not. I headed home and spent the rest of the evening checking my phone, verifying I had a good signal, waiting for the call updating me on Estelle's status.

My phone did not ring the rest of the night or the next day, which was Sunday. On Monday I went to the hospital and discovered that the surgeon on call had performed the surgery early the day before, and Estelle was in the ICU on a ventilator. Because of her advanced age, Estelle was having trouble bouncing back from the surgery. She was my first patient who had more than a simple, everyday illness, and who, despite our best efforts, might not recover. Even though I was aware of the fact my presence would not have changed the outcome, I was still disappointed I had not been called in for the surgery. Perhaps if I had seen firsthand how the procedure progressed her deterioration might not have been as difficult to process.

I checked on her every morning for a week without fail, even if my preceptor had instructed me to be at the clinic rather than the hospital to start the day. I would leave Alex's house early to drive to the hospital to review her chart and perform a cursory exam before going to the clinic. Each day she seemed to get a little worse. Most mornings I would enter her room and find her boyfriend, a gentleman in his late seventies who wore a cowboy hat everywhere but indoors, sitting at her side. Each morning he sat there with tears in his eyes, holding her hand, softly speaking into her ear. I would remind him who I was and ask how she was doing. Without fail he would rise and, while slowly rotating his cowboy hat in his hands, say the same thing every time, "She had a rough night, but she's hanging in there."

This was true until June 6, 2009, when I entered the room and she was gone. She did not die of peritonitis but of the pneumonia that followed her surgery. Intubation is necessary for the sedation required to perform intra-abdominal surgery, and the older and sicker you are the more fluid accumulates in your respiratory system. The more fluid that builds up there, the more likely that your lungs will develop an infection. She did develop an infection, and she did not get better. Unexpectedly, the Corn Nuts she had eaten a week prior turned out to be both one of her last meals and a major contributor to the end of her life.

It was hard not to pull for her as I left her room each morning and to hope that the next time I saw her she would be breathing on her own, that her white blood cell count would have indicated the antibiotics were working, and the infection was clearing. Each day I listened to her lungs I hoped the fluid rattling around in them would be gone. I knew that it would not be easy to recover from a ruptured diverticulum and pneumonia when you are eighty-three years old. I knew, but in the medical textbooks you buy on campus they don't tell you how to let people die, only how to treat their illness. When these treatments fail, it is never easy on those who have been caring for the patient. Some say that the training doctors and physician assistants receive breaks us, that it somehow lessens the emotions we feel when we lose one of our patients to death because we don't have time to care, we have to dedicate our day to treating the living. I do not personally believe that this is in fact the goal of any aspect of medical training, nor even close to being a reality. I believe, instead, that we are taught to eliminate our external reactions and to move on quickly after these losses so that we can give the next patient our undivided attention. The fact remains, that before you develop this ability, you have to lose your first patient to know the emotions involved and how to best work through them so that moving on is possible.

Even though I was not present when the family decided to extubate Estelle and remove her breathing tube, I will never forget her. It is a different kind of sadness when you only briefly know someone before they die, and were tasked with preventing their death. You don't have years of memories to reflect on. If anything, the sadness is different due to the brevity of the time you spent with the patient. I only knew Estelle for a week, and a majority of our time together was her dying while I watched helpless. It is sadness not just from losing human life, but also from watching your best efforts fail. The consolation with this case being I was not the surgeon who tried to save her, I was able to distance myself from this aspect of her death, but it didn't really make me feel that much better. I have since been present at the death of a patient after a long illness, and I was as affected as I was when Estelle died. Despite having more experience with death, I will never be able to forget the first time one of *my* patients died. I will always be able to picture an elderly man clutching a cowboy hat, tears in his eyes, whispering into Estelle's ear.

The greatest problem I had with Estelle dying was that my last words to her had been a lie. "We are going to take care of you. I promise." I told her we were just going to run some tests, and that she might need surgery. The doctor told her that she had an infection in her abdomen and needed surgery and that there were risks involved, but without the surgery she would certainly die.

The surgeon said the same thing, and then likely added, "I will do my very best. We will have you back on your feet as soon as we can." Because we want to alleviate our patients' fears we warn them of risks, but judging the exact level of risk of the procedure can be difficult. The risk of the procedure may be moderately high, yet the risk of not doing anything may be even higher. In this case, we paint the most optimistic picture we can about the procedure because it is practically the only option. Often we do not even realize that these words may be the last the patient hears.

Death helps mold the young PA student into a fully-fledged PA, but it takes a lot of work by the living to teach some of the lessons that harden you the most. I was not far into my first rotation before I met my first "seeker." I can say with certainty that interacting with drug seekers has molded me more in my practice than all the deaths combined. There is a new trend in medicine to view pain as the "fifth vital sign" after heart rate, respiratory rate, blood pressure, and temperature. It is very important to assess pain early in the visit and to control it with as much focus as you would a slow heart rate or severe fever. However, pain is subjective and each patient will respond differently to the same injury or illness. For this reason, medical providers must listen to the description the patient gives of their pain in order to treat it. There are people who take advantage of this inability to categorically measure pain to score narcotic pain medications, either to sell or to use recreationally. Even when pain medication is used appropriately, medical providers must use these medications judiciously, since prescribing for too long or at too high of a dose can lead to dependence on, or even addiction to, narcotic pain medications. Regardless of motive, someone who uses deceit in order to acquire narcotic pain medication is known as a "seeker." I will admit that over my short career I have likely denied narcotic pain medication to a patient in real pain, as well as inadvertently dispensed narcotics to a seeker. Unfortunately there is no easy way to tell when you are being conned, so you just have to go with your gut. However, some patients make it very simple.

It was during the week that I was working with Allen, another physician assistant in the practice, that I met this particular patient. Tuesday afternoon was almost Tuesday evening and I was looking forward to wrapping things up and heading home when Allen asked me to evaluate this patient while he caught up on dictating charts from earlier in the day. I entered the exam room, introduced myself and began documenting the gentleman's history. He had been traveling from farther south, but was moving to the area very soon, and so he had come to establish medical care in the community. He did not have any of his medical records available, but was out of his pain medication and after the long drive up, was having severe back pain. He told the story of how, two years earlier, he had crashed his motorcycle into a tree. As a result of the wreck, he had chronic back pain, for which he took tramadol.

I began my physical exam, beginning with his heart and lungs, but eventually moved to examination of his back, which seemed very tender across his lower spine. He had difficulty bending over or to either side due to his pain. I returned to Allen's office, presented the patient to him, and then we returned to the exam room to wrap up the visit and the day. Allen was very open to the patient's needs and the situation he was in, so he gave the patient a prescription for tramadol that would last one week, which would give him time to have his records sent up from his current clinic. I had completely forgotten about the gentleman by the next morning. We had helped him and would watch the fax machine for his records to come in.

On Thursday night I received a call from the emergency department to say that there was a patient who needed to be seen. I was on call with Janet that night, so it was my job to scurry to the ED as fast as possible. With any luck I could assess the patient, formulate a treatment plan, and present both to my preceptor upon her arrival. The nurses told me the patient was a middle-aged male who had chronic back pain, who had driven in from down south today, but had run out of the meds he takes for his chronic pain. They also mentioned that he asked who he would be seeing this evening, and was informed there was a nice PA named Janet on call. He said that sounded OK and he looked forward to meeting her.

The look on his face when I walked in communicated that maybe it wasn't so OK after all. He looked up with a mild grimace on his face, which quickly fell, followed by his entire head dropping. He rose from the table (without difficulty) and walked out of the exam room, down the hall, and out the double sliding doors at the ED entrance. The nurses asked me if he had gotten lost on the way to the restroom. I almost burst out laughing but managed to inform them that I thought maybe he didn't need to be seen after all. When my preceptor arrived she was curious, to say the least. I explained that Allen and I had seen the patient late Tuesday, had given him a script for tramadol that was to last a week, and that he had presented to the ED that evening for more pain medication.

Janet smiled and nodded. "We get more than a few of those, even in small towns like this," she said. "All it takes is a few major highways to bring them in and an ED they can easily find." Of course, had I not been there the plan could have worked: tramadol from Allen, tramadol from Janet. I have no way of knowing how many other providers he had seen after getting a prescription from Allen or how many he would scam in the future. However, since I was there for both visits by luck alone, any plans he had for Chadron fell apart. I did not see him again the rest of my time there, and I doubt that he appeared in the clinic or ED after that.

Covering the ED that summer gave me some excellent experience, much of which became helpful in future rotations, including some ortho experience I gained ahead of time. Chadron State College is one of four or five Division II NCAA sports programs in the state and easily the most northwestern in the state. The annual summer football camp pulls in football players from all over western Nebraska, not only with the hope of winning the state title but, for a few, of meeting with football coaches affiliated with a program they hope to be recruited by and attend after graduation. They play hard and their injuries show it.

I saw at least two concussed patients in the ED that summer who came in because they had "had their bell rung," but to be truthful it was still ringing when I arrived to assess them. I performed a quick assessment of their recognition of person/place/time/location/etc. and tested their long- and short-term memory. Having had two concussions while snowboarding as a CSC student, I could relate; they could not remember where they were, who I was, or the three items I had given them to remember for all of two minutes. We monitored them, sent them back to the dorms to rest, but had to cut their camp short until they had fully recovered.

These patients were a cakewalk compared to the patients with the orthopedic problems. One unfortunate young man came in after an awkward tackle led to a "pop" in his left knee. He was in excruciating pain and was unable to put any weight on the affected leg. I had learned how to do a full exam, but only on my healthy classmates, and so was hoping that, with an actual patient, I would experience one or more of the telltale signs that would confirm a diagnosis of a particular knee injury. No matter where I touched his knee, which direction I moved his lower leg, he screamed out in pain. I didn't know if I could even finish the exam, if only out of compassion and the knowledge that he likely needed an MRI regardless of what I found. Yet I had him sit up, and I finished the exam. The collateral ligaments on the side of his knee seemed fine, though he was less than happy to have them stretched. Then I checked the stability front to back. Pushing back against his posterior cruciate ligament (PCL) felt fine, but pulling forward I could tell quickly his anterior cruciate ligament (ACL) was not.

Despite my findings, I was too scared to tell the patient on the off chance I had performed the exam wrong or was not really feeling what I thought I felt. So I wussed out, waited until my preceptor arrived, and told him behind closed doors what I suspected: a complete disruption of the ACL. The doctor on call that evening had confidence in my diagnosis and compassion for the patient so he performed only a limited knee exam. He agreed there was no stability front to back. The young man was told to rest, ice, compress, and elevate the left knee, and he was given a prescription for a pain pill, crutches, and told that over-the-counter ibuprofen would not be a bad idea. As soon as he got back to his primary care provider (PCP), the doctor told him, he should ask about an MRI and a referral to orthopedics. In the emergency room it is all about treating the acute injury, but the long-term cure is in some cases left for another doctor down the road.

There are other times in the ED where the treatment has to be very quickly administered for the best possible outcome, as in the case of a shoulder dislocation. Admittedly, it is possible to reduce a dislocated shoulder well after the fact, but it is much easier to accomplish if done within minutes. If there is an athletic trainer on the sideline or another skilled person close by, on-the-scene treatment is optimal. There had been no skilled individuals on the field the evening I was beckoned to the ED for a softball league player who had injured himself sliding into home plate. Upon my arrival, the young man was guarding his right arm, bracing it in his left, and trying to keep the arm from hanging even the slightest, because to do so led to a great deal of pain. I introduced myself as a student and asked him to explain what happened. "Well I was on third base with one out, this girl at bat got under one into right field so I tagged up and headed home. My buddy Steve was the catcher and as I came in I caught his foot with my shoulder and I think it popped out. Ever since then it has hurt like hell."

I asked what I thought was the obvious question: "Were you safe?"

"Hell yeah I was!"

I was afraid he was going to forget he was holding one injured arm with the other and high-five me, but he was in enough pain to remember to sit still. The nurses thought this was a funny question to ask, but I added, "Well if you are going to pop a shoulder out, you have to score the run."

I performed a limited exam because it was obvious the shoulder was dislocated. I felt safe calling in X-ray before my preceptor arrived in order to confirm the dislocation, that there was no fracture, and the direction of the dislocation: anterior/frontward, which is most common, verses posterior/backwards, which is rare. When Allen arrived, he was glad to have the patient off to X-ray. He listened to my presentation of the patient and asked the nurses to call in his supervising physician so that we could use sedation to relocate the shoulder. There are various ways to place the head of the humerus back into the glenoid of the scapula where it belongs in normal anatomy and each requires a different kind of anesthesia. The simplest is to inject local anesthesia medication into the joint prior to manipulation. The problem is that the patient stays alert and aware of everything, and can tense up, leading to difficulty in shoulder relocation. There is complete anesthesia, which is limited to severe cases where it may be necessary to surgically reduce the dislocation. Somewhere in between lies the preference of my preceptor and his supervising physician: sedation where patients continue breathing on their own but they are not aware of the pain, and if they experience any pain, it is quickly forgotten and so it is not a traumatic experience. It is almost like taking a nap that is difficult to arise from, which is good, because reductions are not fun.

When the doctor arrived, the X-rays were readily available and it was confirmed that the patient had not suffered any fracture. He had dislocated his shoulder, and it was anterior in nature, meaning the head of the humerus was in front of the scapula instead of seated in the glenoid where it belongs. We headed back to the exam room, explained the procedure to the patient, and obtained permission to use sedation to accomplish it. The patient was laid on his abdomen, the sedation was administered, and he quickly slipped into a snoring slumber. The affected arm was dangled off the edge of the table and with increasing pressure I was instructed to gently pull the arm towards the floor. This did not elicit much success, likely due to the fact that too much time had passed between the injury and our attempt. A five-pound weight was brought into the room and tied in a towel, which was then tied to the patients drooping arm. The doctor advised me we would wait for the muscles that had tightened up and were inhibiting our progress to tire and allow for reduction. Every five minutes I applied more pressure, and the doctor would press the humerus from above, attempting relocation. After half an hour we continued with the weight, my added pressure downward, the doctor manipulating the scapula from behind, and Allen adding pressure to the humerus of the patient's upper arm.

Finally, after countless attempts, a few seconds into our attempt at pushing/pulling/sweating there was a satisfying "pop!" The shoulder joint had properly relocated. My preceptors stepped back, I removed the weight, and we gently rolled the patient onto his back. The nurses propped the back of the bed up a bit while Allen showed me that although shoulder slings appear simple when on the patient, they come in pieces, and with extra parts out of the box. At least the instructions were not in Swedish like at Ikea. I placed the shoulder sling on the patient and we monitored him in the ED and in X-ray while a post-reduction film was performed. Another half an hour in the ED, with the X-ray showing the reduction had been successful with no new fracture, gave enough time for the patient to awaken enough to be discharged. He was wheeled out to his car (where a friend waited to drive him home), pain medication script and referral to orthopedics in hand. It was my first rotation and I was already getting experience in orthopedics.

The reason I started in family practice for my rotations was so I could "see a little bit of everything." This was most certainly true for my visit to Chadron. Not only did I learn a few things about orthopedics first hand, I also learned how to sew lacerations, remove foreign bodies from eyes/ears/noses, remove skin lesions, and perform a physical exam on actual sick people. Sewing lacerations was by far my favorite; I think that is the case for many students. There is great satisfaction in taking a jagged dirty wound and turning it into a well-approximated, clean, healing line with little threads poking out. My favorite laceration from the Chadron ED came one evening as Alex and I watched the playoffs at our friend Dan's house. I could see it coming minutes ahead not only because the game was tight with the score tied winding down to the last minutes, but also since I could hear the ambulance sirens off in the distance. "Well I might as well head to the hospital and save the rush."

Sure enough, when I was a few blocks from the hospital my phone rang. "We have a sixty-three-year-old female here in the ED, finger laceration with a kitchen knife." At this point in time I figured that this was surely not the ambulance I had heard, but maybe the EMTs had called ahead about that patient as well.

"What about the ambulance? Do we know what they are bringing us?" The nurse on the phone seemed confused, but then understood I was the one who was not following along.

"She came via ambulance."

This struck me as a bit odd, so I double checked just in case "For a finger laceration, not, like multiple fingers, or a hand gash?"

The nurse confirmed that it was a single digit. "It's the thumb on her left hand, but yes, just the one." I decided to give the patient the benefit of the doubt, that driving with a towel wrapped around one hand would prove to be very difficult and she had not been able to reach friends or family to assist her. When I arrived I met the nurses in the ED and found my patient on the bed with a white blood-soaked towel around her left thumb. I introduced myself and asked her if she could tell me how her injury occurred.

"Well I recycle my bottles and I was removing the plastic ring from a Coke bottle with a steak knife when I slipped and stabbed myself right in the thumb."

The nurses had already reviewed her medical history with her, and I saw it had been over ten years since her last tetanus vaccine. "You haven't had a tetanus shot since 1998?"

"Nope."

"No problem there. I bet we can get you one this evening." After Janet arrived, I presented the patient to her, including her need for a tetanus booster. "Wait a minute . . . that was the ambulance?" At least I wasn't the only one who thought that was interesting.

"Yes, she came via ambulance."

Janet frowned, but then was strictly business as usual. "I see. Well the lidocaine is in the back cabinet, the nurses will get you the needles and syringe, I will track down the suture tray . . . wait if she came via ambulance how is she going to get home?"

I told her it didn't come up.

"Well we will find someone to come get her. I know the ambulance doesn't do round trips." Janet went to find the suture tray and I went to find the lidocaine. I drew up about ten milliliters of lidocaine, switched to a smaller needle, and carried it over to the patient. The nurses had gotten my soapy water, Betadine and sterile gauze pads. I put on gloves, cleaned the wound with warm soapy water and Betadine, and inspected the wound for pieces of Coke bottle and to make sure that a simple suture would be adequate to close the wound—that deep closure was not necessary. It was still oozing some blood, but was not so deep that more than three or four superficial sutures would be necessary to close the wound. Then I had a decision to make: I could inject into the laceration itself, or I could place a digital block by injecting around the nerves at the base of her injured thumb. I recalled that placing a digital block on thumbs and big toes can be difficult and figured this was not the time for me to learn why this was the case. I injected into the wound and the lady almost hit the roof, cussing like I had not heard for a long time. I explained that I know the poke hurts, but if you can bear with it, just like at the dentist, it will quickly go numb and the pain would subside. She cussed me one more time and informed me she would try harder.

Second time was a charm and I injected the lidocaine. I inspected the wound a little more and then washed my hands in preparation for the real work. I put on my sterile gloves while the nurses opened up the suture tray, and Janet hovered close enough to see everything but not contaminate anything sterile. I placed small blue towels around the lacerated thumb and clamped them in place with hemostats. Gingerly I removed the needle with suture from its paper wrapping with my forceps and placed it in the grip of the needle driver. I pinched the edge of the laceration with my forceps just to make sure it was numb, and I began the simple closure. Gently, slowly, I pushed the needle through one side of the laceration, under the flap of the opposite side and back through to the surface. I tied it off in the same fashion I had learned sewing up chicken legs and oranges back in Lincoln. Four sutures later the laceration was closed. Now, if she'd had any desire to be a hand model, I was not the best person to help her, but, all things considered, this thumb did not look too bad. It was certainly better than when she brought it to me. Via ambulance.

I am happy to report that during the rest of my family practice rotation in Chadron I did not lose any more patients, nor did I experience any drug seekers, though, as I previously pointed out, some people are excellent actors and I may have been deceived. My sewing skills improved over time, and I also honed my exam skills, learned how to write progress notes, write prescriptions, and order the right test at the right time. I was by no means ready to run out and get a job when I left, but I was no longer a rookie in medicine. I could manage the slightest of medical conditions, and I no longer froze at a patient's door trying to remember as much as possible about their possible condition based on my book knowledge, so that I could be a step ahead during the interview. I now felt confident enough in my own abilities to think on my feet and access that knowledge if I found that my brain did not contain all the necessary information just yet. I was able to use that as a launching point to further my education and learn more about that which I did not know. This was most certainly a good thing, because coming up next was my rotation in surgery with a doctor well known on campus for his abilities to pimp a student into an absolute wreck. This is not as inappropriate as it sounds. It means to ask difficult questions in front of a group of medical professionals, making you look foolish if you cannot answer or answer incorrectly. I hoped I had accumulated a wealth of knowledge during my didactic phase and first rotation, for into the cross-hairs I went.

Surgery
York, Nebraska

My second rotation was in York, Nebraska, just down the road from Lincoln, with two general surgeons at the community hospital. I wanted to be readily available for any emergency procedures, such as appendectomies, and since surgery sometimes started as early as 7:30 a.m. (and not necessarily in York), I stayed in the student housing across the street from the hospital during the week and went home on weekends.

For my first two weeks, I joined Ann, a first-year medical student (M1) who was just wrapping up her surgery rotation, and spent my last two with a different M1. They were as different as day and night, at least on the surface. Ann was intelligent but quiet, either by nature or by nature of having spent two weeks with Dr. Phillips, our preceptor. Tom was confident, but allowed his confidence to get the best of him when it came to the pimp sessions. Though Tom was also in his first year of medical school, Dr. Phillips saved all the anatomy questions for him. In my third year of PA school, I was a good year-and-a-half removed from my last anatomy lecture. I was more than happy to let him handle the odd triangles of hernia repair and suspensory ligaments of the pelvic floor while I fielded the clinical questions. Ann had already proven herself to Dr. Phillips in her first two weeks, and so it was up to me to prove myself in my first two weeks as well. With her help on some of the questions she had already worked her way through, I was in Dr. Phillips's good graces in no time. There were actually two surgeons in the group, the second being Dr. Phillips's partner, Dr. Thornton. A majority of the time was spent with Dr. Phillips, and he certainly enjoyed teaching, as long as you put forth the effort he expected in order to learn.

Surgery in the outlying hospitals was especially fun for Dr. Phillips, as this gave him up to an hour-and-a-half on the road, with no radio, to question and teach us about various disease processes. I took the back seat as much as possible, with all my pocket guides and palm pilot in my lap out of view. I learned this little trick from Ann during our first two weeks. I thought she was just letting us guys sit up front together, but later learned that back there you could only be seen in the rear-view mirror and if you were stumped you could possibly find the answer in your white coat pocket. Also helpful in preparing for these sessions was the fact that my room at the dorm was one of the few that were able to pick up the Wi-Fi signal from the hospital. Thus, I was at an advantage as far as being prepared for the intraoperative quiz sessions my preceptor was known for, because if it wasn't in my books it was certainly somewhere online. I not only had my books but also the World Wide Web at my fingertips to access as much information about the next day's cases as I could. Tom was a little too far out of range and more than once forgot to look up the question he had missed in surgery that day. Somewhere out there are two doctors who helped me breeze through my surgery rotation; one through her share of knowledge, the other through his lack thereof. This is assuming Tom shaped up and graduated.

My favorite pimping story was during the first two weeks when Ann was there to tell me of some of Dr. Phillips' favorite topics, including "Luminal Obstruction!" We were driving up to one of the smaller outlying communities for a day of colonoscopies when Dr. Phillips perked up in the front seat next to me. "Now, Ann, I know you already know all this so you just keep quiet back there. Sean, what is the cause of appendicitis?"

I thought for a bit about the pathophysiology because that was the answer I was going to give, but thanks to Ann I knew where the conversation was actually headed. "An inflamed appendix, which results in infection."

"Ah, yes" Dr. Phillips grinned, "but how does it get inflamed?"

Not wanting to give away the fact that I had been prepped and thus show my hand, I thought a bit more. "Well, the appendix is much like a very large diverticulum, so it gets infected much like a diverticulum would. It is OK for fecal matter to flow in and out, but if it gets stuck the bacteria proliferate."

"Good, you are getting there, but what are appendices? What are diverticuli in their essence?"

I played dumb a bit longer. "Little pouches. Pouches only have one way in or out."

"Yes, but what would be a good term for that condition? What is the lining of a tube or pouch called?"

"You mean like a lumen?" I could almost hear Ann cracking a smile in the back seat.

"Yes, a lumen!" Dr. Phillips perked up in the seat of his Prius. "And what is it called when a lumen is blocked? Ann, you can chime in!"

Ann did chime in from the back. "Luminal obstruction."

"*Luminal obstruction!* And when, say, the gallbladder gets inflamed, then infected, what is it called? Sean?"

"Luminal obstruction?"

"*Luminal obstruction!* And when a sinus is blocked by allergies or a cold, what is the result?"

"Luminal obstruction?"

"*Luminal obstruction!*" This continued for just about every orifice you could imagine getting obstructed, though after he calmed down Dr. Phillips did admit that sinuses are not technically luminal, but they fit in the thought process.

The next two weeks were filled with sessions like this: me answering whatever question Dr. Phillips could think of, either on the spot or taking another shot at the question from the day before if it had been a stumper. Nothing upsets a preceptor more than if you miss the same question twice. Everyone gets one strike at a question, but don't even think about missing twice. Tom did not catch onto this the entire last two weeks of my rotation, which were the first two weeks of his. I recall the two days in a row Tom could not recall the name of the triangle that is bounded by lines joining the anterior superior iliac spine, the pubic tubercle, and the umbilicus. The first day was excusable; the next day Tom was expected to know Sherren's triangle, both inside and out, because on day two he was supposed to name the structures that comprise it. With Dr. Phillips those were strikes two and three all in one whiff.

As much fun as it was learning with Dr. Phillips and the surgical teams we worked with, I must admit there were difficult times. As anyone in medicine can tell you, one of the first things they learned was not to plan on things going perfectly, and to be ready to change things up on the fly. This can be as simple as getting the patient's temperature at the end of the visit and not at the beginning because the patient had just enjoyed a cup of coffee in the waiting room, or as complex as converting a laparoscopic[2] gallbladder removal into an open one. I mention this procedure conversion because I almost viewed this exact occurrence during one of the first surgical cases I scrubbed in on with Dr. Thornton. The intended procedure was a quick in-and-out laparoscopic cholecystectomy to remove an inflamed gallbladder; however, it went on much longer than intended for numerous reasons. The first problem was that in this particular patient the gallbladder itself did not appear as inflamed as the CT scan had initially shown, meaning there was a strong possibility that the problem actually lay above the gallbladder in the common bile duct which carries bile to the gallbladder or the liver itself which produces it. The second

---

2   Minimally invasive surgery performed through small incisions, specialized instruments, and a camera instead of a large incision.

problem was that there were two students taking turns holding the camera for Dr. Thornton during the case. There are two things students do well in surgery: hold retractors during open cases and hold cameras during laparoscopic cases. If it entails standing like a statue for hours, it is just up the student's alley.

The surgery had started at 11:00 a.m. and was expected to take about an hour. However, between passing the camera between students and the non-camera student assisting with an internal retractor, complicated by there being no real cause of pathology, the case took about twice that long. At 12:30 the float nurse in the room asked if maybe the students (Ann and I) should take lunch. Admittedly, this procedure was not going routinely; it was still "just a lap-chole" and there was no reason to starve the students just so they could both watch a simple procedure. We decided Ann could go first and by the time she was done the case likely would be, too. Dr. Thornton explored the common bile duct, found no stone, explored around the pancreas, and explored everywhere until Ann returned. This meant it was my turn for lunch. I was one hundred percent certain by the time I returned the case would be done. I have no idea what I missed, but the case was still ongoing upon my return. So I scrubbed back into the case, and took up my position opposite Dr. Thornton at the table. A few minutes back in, Dr. Thornton had the gallbladder out and was ready to start removing the instruments so we could close the incised areas. Then he nicked the spleen bringing a probe out. The spleen is the most vascular organ in the body, excluding the heart itself. Trauma victims have died from a ruptured spleen, so even a nicked spleen was reason for great concern. The electrocautery probe was quickly inserted back through the largest incision opposite the camera and the nick in the spleen was quickly zapped closed, and though an impressive amount of blood had been pouring out of the affected area, once the cautery had been administered it was probably barely a scratch. The important thing was that disaster had been averted, and the surgery was finally winding down. The instruments were withdrawn for good, the incisions were quickly closed, and the patient was transferred without further incident to the recovery room.

I was getting smarter and more confident as the days went by, and I was certain surgery was the field I wanted to practice in after graduation. It seemed like the perfect life to me, despite the outcome I had with Estelle only a month prior. You walk in, meet the patient, answer a few questions, figure out who the family members are so you can find them afterwards, and off you go. Anesthesia sedates them, you scrub in, prep the patient, cut, fix, off to tell the family of the success. This was true for every inflamed gallbladder we removed, every infected appendix we nixed, and every hernia we sewed mesh reinforcement into. Then came the day we were called to West Bend, an outlying hospital, at about 9 a.m. for an elderly woman with a bowel obstruction secondary to colon cancer. Without surgery she was certain to rupture her intestines into her abdomen and perish within a matter of days, if she was lucky. If she wasn't she would linger on battling sepsis and peritonitis for weeks before she finally succumbed. We began our drive to West Bend and commenced a discussion on what? Why luminal obstruction, of course.

I rested in the back seat, having already passed this little exam, while Tom struggled in the front seat. As long as Tom was the target of the Q and A sessions it was going to be a great day. Upon arriving at the hospital we went straight to the surgery changing area and donned our green scrubs, blue booties, and surgeon caps. We strode down the hall to the patient's room and met Lucy, our seventy-six-year-old bowel obstruction, and her family: two daughters, one son, their three spouses, and two of the grandchildren these unions had brought forth. Like two smug little baby surgeons we watched our mentor feel around on her stomach and chat with the family explaining the procedure. "It is a fairly simple procedure, really. We will open up her belly, find the obstruction in the bowel, and remove it if we can. More than likely this means we will have to place a colostomy with the upper portion to let waste out, and a vent with the lower portion, just to prevent gas building up." It was 10 a.m. when the nurse arrived to wheel her down to surgery.

The three of us—Dr. Phillips and his two little smug shadows who were growing smarter and more confident every day—scrubbed into surgery, backed into OR1, and donned our sterile gowns and gloves. The only downside I could see going into this procedure was that it was an emergent bowel surgery, and so there had not been time for a "bowel-prep" in which GoLYTELY (a misnomer, it should be GoFIERCELY) is given to flush everything out of the intestines, giving a clearer, and thus easier, access to the inner lumen of the colon. Dr. Phillips did what he could to contain the contents, but lest I make you feel queasy, let me just say this: his speed and two suction tubes were not enough to contain the contents. Nevertheless, he was able to remove a good amount of dead bowel and line up a good ostomy site, as well as a vent site just below it. He decided to place the ostomy first, because it was of greater importance than the vent. He allowed both Tom and I a chance to sew the transverse colon into place using a time-tested suture that he had taught us. Next, having mastered this stitch in a matter of minutes, we proceeded to sew the vent site into place.

Easy as pie, time to close, except for one thing: going back up to the ostomy site, it was apparent that for some reason the bowel had continued to die proximal to our site. What was once healthy pink colon was now turning black three centimeters proximal to our stitch site. Dr. Phillips was not pleased to say the least. After three hours of surgery we were at a major setback. We had already given one dose of IV antibiotics; soon it would be time for another. The antibiotic dose was ordered, and the family was told we were still closing but if they liked they should go get lunch and hurry back. A nurse offered to order our lunch since the cafeteria would be closing soon, but there would be no time to eat because an appendectomy waited back in York. We didn't mind because appendectomies are fairly routine and straightforward, and we would eat supper after that procedure was completed.

The now dead tissue was removed from the ostomy site, resected, and a new section, (of ascending colon) was chosen. Halfway through sewing it into place, it became apparent that it too was dying. Dr. Phillips decided to do the only thing possible: cut out the entire ascending colon and place an ileostomy. The entire colon had now been removed, and we were utilizing the small intestine to remove waste from her digestive tract. After another three hours of surgery, we were finally ready to close. Exasperated, Dr. Phillips took what is usually a good sewing practice opportunity for the students and, in the hope of saving time, promptly closed. Lucy was skillfully sewn shut, surgical gowns were removed, and I was handed the chart.

"Get her some more antibiotics and the usual post-op note. Teach Tom here how to do it." Dr. Phillips left OR1 to go into the men's locker room. Me, teach a future doctor? Wait, who said I knew how to write the usual post-op note? Luckily, there was a standard form in the back of the chart. All I had to do was figure out the dosage for the antibiotic.

As I filled this out, the anesthesiologist called us over. "She's not breathing too well on her own."

This was not unusual for an elderly patient after a long surgery; it just meant she needed some time in the ICU on the ventilator. "That's fine. We will just admit her to the ICU and get her on the vent."

I turned back to my note to document this bold decision I was so proud to have made all on my own. "We don't have an ICU, and the ventilator hasn't been approved by the board yet."

I froze. How on earth could we be doing surgery in a hospital with no ventilator? I looked over at Lucy. The anesthesiologist, for some reason, had not re-intubated her, was not bagging her, and for the last minute her oxygen saturation had fallen to 86% (above 90% was normal.)

It was Tom's choice to make the next "bold decision": "Well for the love of God get her intubated then!"

"We can't keep her here in the operating room forever you know." The anesthesiologist seemed to be taking his time finding the right tube, possibly inconvenienced by the notion of intubation.

"I'm going to find Dr. Phillips," I said and started for the door to the men's locker room. Inside, Dr. Phillips was dictating the procedure. "We have a problem. We can't get her extubated."

"Really? That figures. Just our luck. Well get her on the vent. We will have to wean her later."

"They don't have a ventilator. The board hasn't approved it yet."

The next two hours were a blur of activity I cannot even begin to describe. We placed a Swan-Ganz catheter through a major artery in her neck, through her heart, and into her lungs to better monitor her oxygen status. A mobile X-ray unit was brought in to verify the placement was correct. However, we had not planned on intra-operative films so no concern was given to which end of the table the post leading to the floor was on. It was on the wrong side to move in the X-ray machine. Worse yet, despite being intubated, Lucy was still not getting enough oxygen into her body. Four blood gasses were performed, each more difficult than the prior as viable arteries were checked off the list. The problem was that in the eight or so hours since being wheeled into surgery, Lucy's body had become slightly chilled in the sixty-degree operating room, and her vessels had hidden deep in her body to preserve heat.

We eventually were able to get her O_2 saturation above 90% and stabilize her for a flight to Lincoln, where an ICU bed, complete with ventilator, waited for her. In the hospital's defense, the surgery was emergent, was supposed to be simpler than it later became, and a post-op ventilator was indeed in the works, just not on site yet—not that I truly believe an onsite ventilator would have changed anything except the timing. Lucy's heart stopped twice on the helicopter flight into Lincoln and then again on the landing pad of the receiving hospital. The third time was more than she could handle. Eleven hours after we told her that she would be back in her room before supper, eight hours after we told her family that she would be there after their lunch, and four hours after we sewed her shut, Lucy died.

I had now told two people that I was going to help fix them and had failed. We did make it back to York in time to perform the appendectomy before there was a rupture and another case of peritonitis. This was a hollow victory for me. Lucy was the second patient I had lost, but the first one where I had to put my feelings aside and focus on helping someone else. I do not even remember thinking about Lucy during the procedure. She was not on my mind those two times she coded in the helicopter, she was not on my mind as they wheeled her onto the helipad, and she was not on my mind when she died. Instead my thoughts were filled with the procedure at hand: removing an inflamed appendix from a seventeen-year-old. I learned that night to get over death quickly, and to move on: the next patient needed me.

I believed that my next rotation, in obstetrics and gynecology, would be an improvement over my prior rotations, where I had lost a patient on each. Though tales are told of women dying while delivering a child in days gone by, advances have made this a rare occurrence, and so I had no reason to believe that I had any chance of losing another person under my care. Thankfully, this was the case. After spending the first two rotations away from home, only returning home at the end of my first, and only for weekends for my second, it was nice to finally have a rotation in Lincoln. I could finally go home every night and sleep in my own bed.

Obstetrics and Gynecology
Lincoln, Nebraska

My first day in OB/GYN was a smooth segue from my surgery rotation, as I started Monday morning in the operating room for a scheduled caesarean section (C-section). Each rotation was a new start, with a new team, in a new hospital. Despite the fact that I was well versed in sterile technique after my surgery rotation, the surgical nurses kept a keen eye on me for fear I would make a mistake and contaminate the sterile surgical field. I wanted to get off on the right foot with my preceptor, but it is hard to show confidence and skill when everyone around you acts as though they expect you to screw up at any second. Luckily, my preceptor Dr. Wilson was kind from the very start, which made settling in easier. He took time to explain everything to me. However, he did not let me do much more than hold a retractor that first day so I did not get a great view of the procedure, but I did assist in making his view better. After a few C-sections that morning we were off to clinic and the first of many pelvic exams I would either observe or be responsible for.

The greatest difficulty I had during my month in OB/GYN was being male in a clinic consisting entirely of female patients. I fully understand that the examination is guaranteed to make them uncomfortable, no matter who performs it, and that having a male perform it only adds to this discomfort. Though more than once I had to wonder about the thought process when I was dismissed from the exam room for being a man, so that Dr. Wilson, a male, could do it instead. Admittedly, they had seen Dr. Wilson before and had specifically requested his services prior to the visit, and I was a sidekick who just appeared when the visit began. I did learn about establishing rapport with your patients from all of this. A good clinician is not judged merely by who or what they are (e.g., male) but by their actions. Dr. Wilson's patients had grown to trust him, and so were willing to undergo an embarrassing and uncomfortable exam under his care.

I must be honest; I did not enjoy my OB/GYN rotation, and the best aspect of it was that I was able to escape to my own house every evening. There are certain fields of medicine where I cannot help but wonder, "Why would you want to do that all day?" At the top of this list for me is the trifecta of proctology, urology, and gynecology. Don't get me wrong; in most fields of medicine you have to look at an intimate area of your patients, but at least in those you get some visits where patients have their clothes on to mix things up. The lone bright spot of this rotation would certainly have to be the delivery of my first baby. Helping another person bring a child into the world is almost as exciting as seeing one's own child delivered into it.

After two deaths being the strongest memory from my first two rotations, there was no greater joy than experiencing the opposite end of life's spectrum. Unfortunately this joy was staved off at first due to the distance I lived from the OB/GYN clinic and the hospitals where Dr. Wilson had privileges. My phone rang every time one of the clinic's patients was going into labor. The first two times I was disappointed. The first chance I was offered, Dr. Wilson himself barely made it in time to catch the baby, and I was a matter of minutes too late. The second chance I arrived in time to assist in delivery, but the case was not conducive to my participation. As I rushed into the delivery room I was met with a room filled with expectant faces. Right off the bat I felt the stress of delivering a child under such strong pressure. I was not at all relieved to see the nurse midwife had already arrived to monitor the situation until Dr. Wilson and I arrived because of what I saw in her hands. The baby had not controlled his bowels during the early delivery process and had released feces into the birth canal. This first bowel movement is called meconium and its presence in the birth canal is a possible source of infection for the newborn. One cannot be certain that it had been released only moments before and not months before, which meant that I would not be delivering the child since the neonatal resuscitation team would need to sweep him away to the NICU (neonatal intensive care unit) as soon as possible. To say that the meticulous delivery performed by a PA student would have proven to be too much of a delay is a severe understatement. Since we could not prove that the newborn did not have stool in his lungs, I was unable to participate other than by observing the nurse midwife deliver the baby. When Dr. Wilson arrived, he did little more than dictate the care to follow delivery. Luckily, the newborn baby boy was fine and was discharged with only a small delay.

My third opportunity for delivering a child was the charm for which I had been waiting. The call came during clinic hours so Dr. Wilson and I drove a few blocks together, which afforded me enough time to deliver a sixteen-year-old high school student's first child. These first-time moms usually progress through labor slower, and this allows for a good teaching experience because there is time to talk things over, and yet the pelvis is pliable enough to usually allow easy passage for the child. With Dr. Wilson hovering over my left shoulder, he guided me through positioning the child's head as it presented. He helped me suction the baby's airway so she could breathe, the mother gave one final push, there was a gush of the amniotic fluid that had been the baby's cushion in the womb for nine-and-a-half months, and I delivered my first child. I cannot begin to explain the warmth I felt in my heart as I handed the mother her firstborn child, with the father looking on, a glow upon both their faces.

The rotation continued without fanfare after that first delivery. Though I prayed for maybe a little fanfare, in the main hallway of the clinic were photos of a certain Blue Collar Comedy Tour member who had chosen to return to his home-state to birth his babies. If he had walked through the door to say hello, I likely would have fainted. Instead, day in and day out was filled with Papanicolaou smears (or Pap smears) screening for cervical cancer, writing scripts for birth control for embarrassed teenagers and college students and unembarrassed soccer moms, and postpartum visits. At postpartum visits my job was checking for problems that may arise after delivery, such as a uterus that has not returned to its normal non-pregnancy state, screening for signs of infection in the vagina and pelvic organs, and, of course, performing a Pap smear. After a successful pregnancy with delivery it has been at least ten months since the last Pap, and since they are performed on an annual basis anyway: two birds with one stone.

Now, I have already mentioned that this rotation was not all butterflies and jellybeans for me, and I never expected it to be. I just never thought it would cause actual strife in my life, especially as far as my training went. Bouncing from one preceptor to another did not cause any problems when I was in Chadron, but was almost my downfall during this rotation. Dr. Wilson opened his practice with his female cousin, who had been his original PA. Later they added a recent graduate of my own PA program, Sally, who was hired to help as the practice grew. Sally was the preceptor who evaluated me at my mid-rotation evaluation; the one that doesn't count. I knew I wasn't doing fantastically, since OB/GYN isn't exactly my cup of tea, but she told me I was doing fine and not to worry about it. I will say that she did me no favors by letting me slide at the two-week mark, because when it came time for my final evaluation and my grade on the rotation, Dr. Wilson tore me apart. It was quite a gut check to read the evaluation at my first quarterly meeting, especially after getting perfect marks on my first two evaluations. Furthermore, at this quarterly meeting I had already received three As, including a perfect score on OB/GYN prior to receiving my preceptor evaluations. In fact, it was only that perfect score on the written portion that brought my grade for OB/GYN up to a low B and allowed me to continue in the program. Any possibility in my mind that I wanted to practice as an OB/GYN physician assistant (not that there was more than a shred of desire to do so) shriveled up and died as I read the words Sally had spared me from, and that Dr. Wilson himself could not take the time to express to me in person.

You get over these things with time, just as any other bad day in medicine so that you can move forward to the next task requiring your undivided attention. The fact remains that the sting lingers during the immediate aftermath. That would be the summation of my first quarter as a PA student: you can't let the bad things stick with you. You have to move on and take care of the patient in the next room, or, in my case, you have to move onto your next rotation and keep trying to do your best. While OB/GYN did little to win me over, I have to admit that it did help me when my second family practice rotation came up the following winter in my small Nebraska hometown. In communities like these, there are typically no OB/GYNs, just family doctors who wear many hats. Also, I have to admit it was nice to finally spend a month with no one dying.

I know this much for certain: I had only been mildly desensitized to death before this rotation. I fear that if I had lost a mother, her baby, or God forbid both during this rotation I worry I may not have been able to continue my rotations. At least not without a break to process it all. The two patients who had died up to this point were at least elderly. The death of a new mother and/or her newborn itself may have been too much for me. Not only was a break from death welcomed, it was likely necessary for my overall mental wellbeing.

My next rotation was more my speed, and went much more smoothly. This rotation was the one that pulled me in, and ultimately became the field in which I practiced in my first year after graduation. It was also the second rotation in a row I was able to perform in Lincoln, and you cannot put a price on sleeping in your own bed.

Orthopedics/Sports Medicine
Lincoln, Nebraska

The weekend before my first day on my orthopedics rotation, my son came down with a stomach virus and decided to share it with me. I probably would have been fine if Mondays had not been surgical days for the ortho group with which I was to spend the next month. The previous night had been spent in the bathroom suffering miserably, and around 2:30 a.m., driving to a drug store for bismuth sulfate (knock-off Pepto-Bismol). On my first day, a lack of sleep and a whole lot of dehydration bogged me down. Blood and guts, by this point in time, were not bothersome to me, but I had trouble making that known the first day as the room started spinning and a tunnel closed in on my field of vision in the middle of our first case. I quickly notified my MD and PA preceptors of my sudden wooziness, and was escorted to a chair far from the surgical field before I found myself falling face first into it. Dr. Williamson and Chester his PA were friendly guys, but, being orthopods, they of course gave me grief about it. I disclosed that I was living with a vector for just about every virus known to man, and they seemed to understand that I was not truly that faint of heart. Luckily, it was a twenty-four-hour kind of bug and, after scooping myself off the chair in the back of the OR suite, I hit the ground running and both enjoyed and learned much on my rotation despite this first rough day.

My ortho preceptor was a jack-of-all-trades, which was certainly conducive to me learning as much as I could about orthopedics as fast as possible. Normally, my school only required us to spend two weeks on ortho, since we would pick up some sports medicine in other rotations (such as family practice), so once we knew what a joint replacement was and whether or not we enjoyed them, we were scooted off to the next thing. The trick in Lincoln in landing the "good" ortho rotation, and really benefiting from it, was to declare you wanted a two-week Sports Medicine Elective to follow your mandatory ortho rotation. This practice would only take students for a month at a time; no two-weekers were allowed. Only one other PA student in my class lucked into this situation; we both felt like we had found hidden treasure. I have been to a few state meetings in Nebraska, and every year either Dr. Williamson or Chester gave a lecture on one ortho topic or another. These are truly some of the best people I could have possibly learned from. It was a breath of fresh air after my prior rotation, without a doubt.

There is a joke in medicine that the bottom 10% of the class is lobotomized; those who crawl away go into obstetrics and the rest go into ortho. This is likely also the source of the joke that orthopedics is just carpentry. Find bone, measure, cut (the good ones measure twice then cut), hammer in new joint, and sew shut. It is certainly not for the squeamish (or those harboring enterovirus), because limbs are contorted into strange positions when dislocated for a joint replacement, and blood flies with each hammer swing or saw blade movement. I must have been lobotomized well because I took right to it.

Between scheduled knee/hip replacements there were knee and shoulder scopes and the occasional fracture. Fractures were probably the best because of the satisfaction of helping patients in severe acute pain distance themselves from that misery as fast as possible. Admittedly, this was not always the case; if the patient was too old or their heart too weak for surgery the best we could do was line up the bones as close as possible, cast the extremity, and let time heal what it could. When the fracture was an impressive one, and the patient was a good candidate for surgery, we would swoop in, tell the family it would be OK, and make it so. A few hours later we would return having fixed the fracture. I had learned the hard way not to feel like some sort of superhero, but with the success rate Dr. Williamson and Chester had I felt at least a little super being part of their team. It was wonderful that we only had news of success to report after every surgery. Perhaps that is one big reason I enjoyed this rotation so much: no one died.

The most interesting case I recall was one that I never saw go to surgery. It came out of the outpatient clinic, needed surgery, but the surgery was not performed during my ortho rotation. In the clinic we saw a fair number of workers' compensation patients, some truly injured, some with dollar signs in their eyes. We also saw a fair number of people who had just flat out worn out their joints during a life of hard labor. "You need a sit-down job," we would tell the construction workers. "You need a job with less computer work," we would tell the carpal tunnel sufferers.

But occasionally a person with "no known injury" would appear. This meant a thorough history was necessary to tease out the underlying detail. I was given free rein with these patients, in the hopes that my interview would save my preceptor valuable time in the investigation phase of the visit, and let him focus on the treatment details. One such young gentleman came in with no known injury and thigh pain. He was a Mormon missionary, which was important to note because this meant he spent his days walking door to door with his backpack weighing him down for hours on end. This indicated he could have pain due to overuse and just needed a break. He may have caused soft tissue damage tearing a muscle, ligament, or tendon. At the worst, it could even indicate an injury to the bone.

I spent a fair amount of time going over when the pain had started, where it was exactly, what made it better, and what made it worse. With young people there is usually a quick onset of pain that can help explain the injury. With this gentleman, it seemed to have crept up on him. I ordered X-rays (because that is always a good place to start, and they are non-invasive.) The X-rays came back negative, which truthfully was no surprise given his age and story. Since his bones were fine, the next step was to investigate the soft tissues of the affected area, which is best accomplished via MRI. So we ordered an MRI, expecting to find that he had strained a ligament, sprained a tendon, torn a meniscus, or possibly had an ACL injury of one sort or another. However, when the results of the MRI came back, all of these structures were fine.

There was, however, the matter of the football-shaped tumor growing out of the young man's femur (thighbone). We had him scheduled for follow-up later that week, and when he came we told him that it was likely a cystic structure, however we recommended he have an oncologist in the room when the area was opened to examine the growth. He requested his records be sent back to Utah where he had family (can't blame him at all), and so I was not there when they took the tumor out of his leg. It is a bit selfish of me to wish I had been in the OR suite when the surgery was performed. Normally, young healthy men don't grow footballs on their femurs. I wish I had been able to follow that one through and find out what the pathology of his growth showed.

After the fantastic football femur, it was back to workers' comp, sprained ankles, and worn-out hips and knees. It was also about this time I discovered I had no idea how to find my way around the shoulder during arthroscopy procedures (scopes). Many an afternoon was spent looking back and forth between a monitor displaying the inside of the shoulder in question, the outside of the shoulder trying to see exactly where the camera was pointed, and back again. Each structure, though miniscule in size, appears enormous on the monitor, somewhat distorting the anatomy. I had only viewed the inside of a shoulder joint on a cadaver prior to my clinical rotations, and you don't want your face zoomed in too close to a cadaver. Trust me. Sadly, it was not until about two months into my first job later on, that I finally figured out exactly what was going on during a rotator cuff repair. This is certainly strong support for extending the ortho rotation in physician assistant training. It might be carpentry, but when you try to do it through a straw, things get complicated rather quickly.

The arthroscopy repair I remember the most was that of an older female stroke patient who had worn out her good arm pulling herself about her home in her wheelchair. I remember her because of her tenacity. She had already had her right shoulder repaired once, and had already had a right knee replacement. When her shoulder tore the first time, while she recovered she pulled herself about with her right leg, and it then wore out as a result. So she had a total knee replacement on her right knee, and then tore her right shoulder while recovering from that. There was absolutely nothing holding her back. We did advise that she look into an electric wheel chair for future use. I can say without a doubt, that if using the joystick on an electric wheelchair wore out her wrist, she'd schedule the wrist surgery and work that chair with her elbow while recovering.

The fact that Dr. Williamson and Chester do workmen's comp was certainly beneficial to my maturing as a PA student. Most of these patients had fantastic stories about their injury, whether it was falling off scaffolding or being struck by an object (often a hammer, but sometimes another tool, and sometimes off scaffolding), but the ones that made me wince were the ones where the patient got a body part caught between two objects. Most notably a gentleman who had his foot become caught between a pre-fab house and the ground. There were more than a few fractures, but some patients were lucky enough to escape with just a very deep bruise. Dr. Williamson's job was to determine how long the patient would need to recover, when they could be returned to full duty, and just what activities were allowed during light duty. For the most part, a construction worker cannot do anything at work that includes "light duty." They are heavy-duty workers or they stay home. Then there were the cases where either due to too much heavy duty or too severe of an injury, the patient could not recover. In these cases disability was the only option left for the patient. This level of workmen's compensation is fraught with the possibility of abusing the system, and so it took a great deal of evaluation before a patient could be labeled with this status. I cannot recall a single patient who received full disability, but I remember the one who lobbied for it the most.

When I entered the exam room the top of the chart said, "Severe Back Pain; discuss disability." I entered the room and introduced myself to the gentleman in the chair next to the exam table. "Could I have you climb up onto the table and take a seat there?"

He grimaced, rose slowly and climbed up onto the step jutting out of the table, slowly turned around, and gently sat on the white paper covering the exam table. "That sure wasn't easy. Ever since I wrenched my back on that construction site about a year ago, I can't hardly walk."

I reviewed his file and saw that he had been treated by his family doctor for lower back pain, but that numerous interventions had failed. Physical therapy, pain medication, and anti-inflammatory medication—both oral and topical—had failed to provide relief. I also saw that an MRI had shown only a mild change in his spine. "I see here the MRI report talks about a few disks in your lower back that poke out a little bit. Tell me more about your pain."

"Well it hurts to walk, but sitting is a little better. Hard to lie down at night. It is right here." He lifted up his right thigh as he leaned to the left and put his right hand on his lower back. "Goes all the way across to the other side though, all through here."

I made note of this so that I could adequately explain the case to Dr. Williamson. I inquired as to the cause of the pain. "This happened at work when you were stepping down from a fork lift?"

The patient slowly returned his leg to the table with a grimace on his face. "Yep, stepped down and it was like I got shot in the butt and the bullet went right up into my back."

I jotted this information down. "And did it go away, come back, come and go since then? Has it been constant?"

"It went away a little bit, but it is always there."

Eventually, it was time for the exam, which was very standard: palpating the affected area, poking and prodding elsewhere, having him bend at the waist in every direction possible, and a few tricks Chester had taught to identify if a patient is malingering or faking at all. This patient seemed to be exaggerating his pain, at least a little. This is unfortunate because it is patients like this who make getting help more difficult for people with no ulterior motive, who are only hoping to escape their real pain. I exited the room and explained everything to Dr. Williamson, including the reservations I had.

Of course, Dr. Williamson could not just take a PA student's word for it, so my entire interview and physical exam was repeated, with no change whatsoever. Dr. Williamson explained to the patient that there was certainly something going on, and perhaps repeating the MRI would be beneficial to glean more information, especially if something had changed since the last one had been performed. I felt a rush of warmth go over me, because I had been ready to dismiss the patient as a malingerer and here Dr. Williamson was proceeding to investigate his pain. The patient was told the imaging department would call him to set this up soon, he was told to follow-up after the MRI, and sent on his way. My embarrassment faded quickly when Dr. Williamson told me to follow him and crept toward the lobby after the patient. The patient limped slowly out to the receptionist, told her he would have the MRI sent over from the hospital when it was done, and limped out the front door. Dr. Williamson crept into the lobby, just far enough to see out the front window. Over his shoulder I saw what he saw: our patient limped to the last row of cars, and when he thought he was out of view, he stopped limping, took a few normal strides to his car, and slid in without difficulty.

"You always give them the benefit of the doubt, then investigate thoroughly to see if the story matches the pain and the pain matches the exam."

I nodded in agreement as he added, "And *always* watch them walk out to their car." Sage advice from one of my favorite preceptors; I had certainly learned a lot in just four short weeks.

Internal Medicine
Grand Island, Nebraska

After finishing up in ortho, it was time for me to travel to the middle of the state to one of the Veteran's Association hospitals in Grand Island for my Internal Medicine rotation. There are VA hospitals closer to my school—the closest is in Omaha—but when it comes to selecting rotations it is first-come-first-serve, so I was placed in the second-closest VA hospital. This facility served all of western Nebraska, but also took overflow from the Omaha VA when there were no available beds. This rotation was about ninety miles from Lincoln, which meant I was back to living in the student dorm all week and returning home only on weekends. I did take solace in knowing that this was my last dorm rotation. Unfortunately, I did have two more rotations that would keep me from my own bed, but at least these would allow me to stay with friends or family.

Up to this point I had been to a clinic this size, but had not yet been to a medical center that served so many in such a large campus. There were five or six floors, most of which were specialty clinics, but one was an inpatient floor that served as a skilled nursing facility for local United States military veterans. Should a patient on this floor become too ill for the level of care provided at the VA skilled care, they were transported out to a community hospital nearby. It was on this inpatient floor that I started every morning, rounding with Julie, an Advanced Registered Nurse Practitioner (ARNP), a pharmacist, a pharmacy resident, and two pharmacy students who were staying across the street with me in the student housing.

Every day we began by checking on the patients under the care of the ARNP. There were many patients on skilled care, all of whom needed many providers to properly care for them, to assess the care they were receiving, and to coordinate their care. It was here that I fully began to appreciate the health-care team mentality of patient care. Julie and I would assess overall status, wound care, nutritional status, etc., and at appropriate times the pharmacy people would add their input as to medicine changes and suggest dosage changes based on symptoms. The most valuable input pharmacy was able to provide was in regards to changes in insulin dosage, since most of the patients under our care were diabetic and had problems with blood sugar control.

After these morning rounds, it was time for me to grab a quick bite to eat and then go to see patients with a number of physicians and PAs in an outpatient clinic. This clinic was more or less the same as a family practice clinic, with the exception that a majority of the patients were over fifty and none were children. As such, I spent a great deal of time in clinic treating the early-disease aspects of disease processes I had just discussed earlier in the day at the skilled care facility: diabetes, hypertension, hyperlipidemia, and arthritis. In fact, one could easily see some of these outpatients becoming residents upstairs in only a few years if we were not successful in slowing down their disease processes.

I was assigned three patients to manage during my month at the Grand Island VA: one who died while I was there, one who wished he could die, and one cancer patient who would die slowly after I had left to continue my education elsewhere. It was the last who was the hardest to see each day because nothing I did would improve his health. The first patient, the one who died under my care, was approaching death due to very advanced stage heart disease. His critical state was almost fully due to his refusal to take his Lasix. Lasix is a drug that helps in heart failure by moving the fluid that accumulates in the body as a result of the blood's sluggish journey through the vascular system with no good pump to keep it in a strong motion. I was assigned the task of acquiring a history and physical on him for his admission to our facility. One could argue that he was a strong candidate for the community hospital, but his non-compliance and failure to follow orders meant he would not benefit much from their care. He could refuse his drugs just as easily at the VA hospital as he would at the outlying facility.

After we had wrapped up joint rounds, I made my way back to the floor and entered his room. "Good morning, Mr. Albertson. I am Sean, a PA student. I will be getting the ball rolling on your admission to the VA this morning."

"I'm not taking the damn Lasix!"

I could tell already this was going to be a fun admission. "Alright, but it looks like you are on a number of other medications. Let me just go over those and make sure we have them all."

"If it's on that sheet it's right!" Nothing like a grumpy guy right before lunch. The transfer paperwork appeared complete, and since he was so pleasant I decided to just move on to the physical exam. The nurse had arrived with the thermometer and pulse-oximeter to check his oxygen saturation, so I gave her the patient's right side, while I moved over to his left. I started to listen to his heart as the nurse took his blood pressure.

"Do you have to pump that thing up so tight?!"

Let me tell you, I definitely heard that one loud and clear. The nurse popped one ear of her own stethoscope out of her ear, "If you took your Lasix and lisinopril, Mr. Albertson, your blood pressure wouldn't be so high and I could start at a lower pressure, but since you don't, here we are." She popped the stethoscope back into her ear. I assumed from the scowl on his face he had nothing to add on the matter, and since my hearing was almost back to normal, I returned to my exam. I listened to his heart, and was glad I gave it another try. I had been through all of the online training modules back in Lincoln during the didactic phase of my education. I had heard a few benign heart murmurs prior to this (the ones where you ask the patient, "Have you ever been told you have a heart murmur?" and they confirm that they have, and it has been there ever since they can remember). I had heard a few stiff valves in older patients, where the blood going through the opening makes a harsher sound than normal. I had even heard a few valves that didn't close completely, allowing a "whoosh" during one phase or the other of the "lub-dub" sequence.

This was my first experience with "Tennessee." Normal hearts go "lub-dub." Sometimes there will be a split in the "lub" as two valves in the heart close not quite at the exact same moment. But when you get an extra sound, it means there is a sick heart under your stethoscope. A third heart sound can be heard in very fit athletes, pregnancy, or in older people whose hearts are sick and failing. A fourth heart sound (so named because it comes later than the third one described above) is a sign that the heart has failed. The third heart sound, S3, is taught using the mnemonic KEN·tuck·Y because it falls right after the two normal ones, S1 and S2 (lub and dub). The fourth heart sound, S4, is taught using the mnemonic te·NNE·see, and that is what I heard in this gentleman. A failed heart. I moved on to the lung exam, and found the distant moist sounds of a patient whose heart cannot pump strongly and whose lungs are now congested because of the pressure this builds inside the pulmonary system.

I moved on to his abdomen and was pleased to finally find something healthy in my patient. I lifted the sheet to observe his legs and check his distal pulses, and found that open blisters had been oozing fluid over both his shins. I checked his icy cold ankles for pulses and found none. His toes were almost as white as the sheet—a stark contrast to his lower legs, which were bronzed and discolored by pooled blood that had disintegrated years prior. I documented my findings in his chart below where the nurse had placed his vitals: Temp 100.1, HR 80, Resp: 28, BP 200/110, O_2 Saturation 90% on 2L of oxygen via nasal cannula. I noted he was febrile, and knew I would have to find the source of his elevated temperature. I added a urinalysis with culture if the initial findings indicated that he might have a urinary infection, as well as a complete blood count to gain insight into the severity of the infection, if he was mounting a response, if he was anemic, etc., and a complete metabolic chemistry profile, because if we are going to poke him, we might as well get as much information as possible. Besides, he was supposed to be on a diuretic so better check his electrolytes.

I could tell you which of his labs were abnormal, or I could save time by telling you that only his calcium and magnesium were normal. He had protein in his urine—a urinary tract infection, an elevated white blood cell count, and all of his electrolytes were low except his potassium, which was too high. This guy was a train wreck, plain and simple. I did not get these labs until I met with the medical team for rounds the next day. I spent ten or fifteen minutes formulating a plan for him: antibiotics for his UTI/elevated WBC, oral sodium supplementation, Kayexcelate to lower his potassium, and now that he was on IV Lasix he would probably need daily electrolyte checks.

When my preceptor arrived, I dived right into presenting this game plan to her while she looked for the patient on our round list. "He isn't on the list. Let me call down to the floor." Moments later she informed me that although my plan sounded excellent, it was all for naught. The patient had passed away early this morning. I folded up my notes on him and tossed them into the shred box under her desk. All that hard work with hopes of improving his condition, adding days to his life, and perhaps decreasing his suffering as well failed to come in time. I got over this death very quickly, either because I only met him the day before or because by now I had faced death before. Mostly, his death did not upset me because he didn't take care of himself, didn't listen to his doctors. Quite frankly, when you are as sick as he was, if you don't take your pills, you die.

The second inpatient I was assigned to during my IM rotation was a Korean War veteran who had had a rough course of pneumonia and had bounced back and forth between the community hospital and our inpatient floor. When I met Robert he was exhausted, could barely breathe, and every second of his life was agony as he fought to exchange carbon dioxide for oxygen. His family was by his side, and immediately his daughter took a firm grasp of my hand and thanked me for coming so quickly. I could tell promptly that my preceptor had given me this patient for two reasons: to teach me about family dynamics, and so that I could take the time and effort necessary to work through them while she tended to more pressing matters.

"It is just so wonderful to have Daddy back here at the VA. This place feels more like home, and I know he will do much better here."

I reviewed Robert's chart and saw that the doctors at the community hospital had found bacteria, specifically Streptococcus pneumoniae in Robert's lungs. I saw that he had initially responded well to antibiotics, but his respiratory function had decreased despite normal blood counts and nothing abnormal in his sputum. "It looks like they got his infection cleared up rather well, but his lungs still aren't that great."

His daughter moved quickly to hold her father's hand. "Oh, I know, but now that we are back here I just know he will get better."

I reviewed the new medications Robert had been placed on, the various nebulizers to mist the medicine into his lungs, percussion of the lung fields throughout the day to break up the congestion, oxygen to keep his O_2 saturation in the normal range, and rescue inhalers when he felt that all this was not enough. "To tell you the truth, looking at his chart he is on just about every respiratory drug known to man. I tell you what, though. I will look into it some more, and see if there is anything I am not thinking of, and what the most recent studies show might be the next step."

Plato said a wise man knows that which he does not know, so I did not feel foolish taking some time to research the case. I consulted my favorite website, which is always up to date on the latest recommendations. However, all I could really find was that we could go higher on the dosage of a few meds, and we could schedule some of his medications slightly more frequently, but not much, and with risk of the side effects outweighing any benefit. By the time I was able to return to Robert's room it was empty except for him. His eyes shot wide open, and I could tell he wanted to talk to me as his shaky hand rose from his bed in my direction.

"Hello, Robert, sorry for the delay. Even worse, I am sorry to tell you we could maybe increase your medications a little bit, but you really are on an impressive cocktail of medicine."

His eyes grew moist, and he placed his hand on mine as I arrived at his bed rail. Through speech broken by his difficulty breathing, the hiss of the oxygen flowing through his mask, and tears in his eyes, Robert told me what he could not tell his family. "I am so tired of all this. I can't do it anymore. This has to be worse than drowning. I can't catch my breath. Ever. I can't hardly move without getting winded. I don't want to live like this. I want to go. I can't take it anymore." He panted beneath his oxygen mask, and gripped my hand tighter. Robert wanted me to be his voice, for I had the breath behind it. It was then that I realized that Robert, if only a little stronger, could have had this discussion with his daughter. If he had tried in his present condition, by this point in time, when she would surely be placing her rebuttal before him, he was too spent to speak again.

I set his chart on his bed and placed my free hand on top of his. "I understand completely Robert and I don't blame you. I know that you likely felt this way before today, but in light of what I just told you, there is a strong argument for not doing anything heroic the next time you catch pneumonia. Honestly, with the congestion in your lungs, it is only a matter of time—perhaps weeks—before you get sick again. Bacteria love a warm, moist environment and that is just what your lungs provide."

Robert nodded, and a tear streamed out of each eye. "Thank you," he wheezed quietly.

As I exited his room, I told the nurses that when the family, specifically his daughter, returned, to page my preceptor so she could find me and we could have a discussion together. Also, if they didn't show up before I left at five, to please call them and see if they would be available sometime tomorrow.

After that I scurried to Julie's office to get her up to speed on my discussion with Robert. "I don't blame him either, Sean. That man has bounced back and forth like a ping-pong ball. Hell, I don't even know how he survived getting out of the hospital bed, into the transport van, and upstairs into our facility this time."

The family did not appear that day, but were at the bedside when the entire medical team rounded the next morning. It had been decided, since I had had the discussion with Robert, that I would open, but since my preceptor was the actual provider and familiar with the family, she would step in shortly thereafter.

We entered the room and I greeted him. "Good morning, Robert. How are you this morning?"

The daughter was already at his side, stroking his forehead. Robert shook his head. "Oh, Daddy is having another rough day, but I know we can get through it. The nurses told me you were going to change his medications so he could breathe better."

I opened Robert's chart so I could list the medications we could maybe alter, if that were decided by the family. "Well there are a few we could change, and that will possibly help for a short period of time, but I don't think they will cure anything, and I don't think there is anything we can do, honestly, that will get him back to where he was before this most recent transfer out for pneumonia."

His daughter looked lovingly back at her father. "Well, every little bit helps. Right, Daddy?" Robert's eyes spilled over.

I knew now was the moment that if he were able to he would tell her, and so I did. Addressing the daughter, her husband, and their children, I explained the discussion from the day before. "I spoke with your father, your grandfather, yesterday, and explained that though we can change his meds ever so slightly, that this will not make any great improvement in his ability to breathe. Also the congestion, the tightness in his lungs will not go away. Ultimately, this atmosphere in his lungs is ripe for another infection to move in."

I paused to let that sink in and Julie, sensing my next sentence, jumped in at that time. "That is correct. I have reviewed Robert's chart, and yesterday afternoon I spoke with Robert myself. He told Sean yesterday morning, and told me later, that when he gets sick again he doesn't want to transfer out for acute care, and he doesn't want antibiotics here. He just wants to be as comfortable as possible."

This code phrase, some people get, others don't. In fact, I have met numerous people who don't like to say "as comfortable as possible" because it doesn't convey the brevity of that situation.

The daughter did not understand completely. "But if he gets an infection he *needs* antibiotics, otherwise he might die." By now I was worried that Robert was going to get too runny of a nose to breathe properly, even with his mask, which was fogging up from the extra moisture his tears were creating.

He managed to speak quietly. "Samantha, I don't want to live like this. It's been a good fight."

"But, Daddy . . ." This was too much, and the daughter began crying, pulling both of her father's hands into hers.

My preceptor stepped closer, placed one hand on Robert, one on his daughter. "This isn't an easy decision for Robert, but he has thought about it long and hard. He doesn't want you and the grandchildren to have to see him like this, and there is almost no hope of making him better. I understand this is difficult news to take, but don't worry because Sean and I will keep an eye on him and make sure he is doing OK. We just aren't going to do any more grand measures if a big problem arises."

By this point, the daughter had shut us out. Her husband stepped to her side and placed his arm around her. "It's OK, honey. In fact, it is better that we get to ease into this idea. I mean he is doing OK, so we get to enjoy these 'OK days' with him, and when things get worse we will know what that means. It has to be better than getting hit out of the blue with it." The room filled with the silence, broken only by her sobs. The husband peered over his wife. "Thank you for taking time to talk to us today. How about you give us some time to process, and if we have any questions we will ask the nurses to get hold of you?"

"That sounds fine. Feel free to ask anything, anytime." Julie escorted the team out the door.

I can tell you that it is never easy when you have to tell a patient that nothing more can be done to prolong their life. If the patient initiates the discussion, it is slightly easier—at least you don't have to break the news to them. When Robert told me he was ready to die, I believed him and would have done nothing spectacular to prevent his demise. He would have wanted it that way. Francis was different. The entire time I spent with him at the VA was to "keep him as comfortable as possible." This was almost like saying, "we can't save your life, but we can make death hurt a little less," which is little solace if you ask me.

Francis was initially just like the others, a new patient whose story needed to be investigated, a task easily handled by the student. Francis was being transferred from the Omaha facility because of the end-of-life, or palliative, care provided by the Grand Island facility on its inpatient floor. He was suffering from pancreatic cancer following a tumor resection known as a Whipple procedure (or pancreaticoduodenectomy, my two favorite medical terms to say out loud, but my least favorite to actually encounter) six years prior. The survival rate for pancreatic cancer following a Whipple resection is around 20% at five years, so this gentleman was lucky to have made it as long as he had and he certainly knew it. As we progressed through his history and physical exam, he was the most stoic person I had ever met—and still is.

He was a Korean War veteran and almost looked the stereotypical part, like Tommy Chong but much thinner, and he was much more reserved. I could not tell if it was the army man in him or the cancer victim facing his mortality that made him as stoic as he was. We went over all his transfer meds, including his Creon tablets, which he would ask for on schedule like a heroin addict sticking to his methadone regiment because he knew that without this drug he would suffer terrible gastrointestinal distress.

"So you had the Whipple in 2004? And it seems as if they got the entire tumor, clean borders on the pathology report."

He let his head drop a bit, letting the stoicism fade away. "Yeah they got it, and that got me more years than I expected, but . . ." He trailed off and looked out of the one window in his room.

"All things considered, someone did something right to keep you up and running this long. It was about the time that you retired?"

He looked back at me, then down at his hands. "Yeah, I used to work at the Henry Doorly Zoo there in Omaha. My job was to keep the penguin exhibit nice and clean, front and back. You can see the penguins up front by the glass, but back behind we have to keep their food fresh, maintain the refrigeration units. Hell, I think there is more behind that wall than in front." For the first time he smiled, half with pride for his years of service and the other half recalling just how much work had gone into it. I have been to the Omaha Zoo at least a dozen times. My favorite exhibit is the Desert Dome, but prior to its construction my favorite was probably the jungle. In times like this, a small fib can bridge a great distance between two strangers.

"You kept the penguin exhibit up and running? That has got to be my favorite part of the Henry Doorly Zoo. I could sit there and watch those guys all day: jump into the water, swim around, jump out, repeat."

His smile grew. "Yeah my granddaughter loved it, too. She said it looked like they were running around in little tuxedos." Then his face fell and tears filled his eyes. "I hope Susan can find the time to bring her down here before . . ." His gaze returned to the window as he wiped the tears away and added, "Well maybe I will get back to Omaha. I'm just here due to crowding at their VA."

I had hoped to cheer him up, to find a connection with him, and likely I did, but when you are facing the end of your life, death looms behind everything. It can even hide behind the happiness. The penguin exhibit with his granddaughter is quickly twisted into: I hope I can see her again before I die. I did not have the heart to tell him the fear in my mind that he would never see Omaha again.

This concern about never seeing his granddaughter again was very valid. During my stay with Francis (as he was still alive when I had to move on to my next rotation) I did not see his daughter or his granddaughter once, due to the distance and their schedules in Omaha. I distinctly remember the day that started with a family meeting, via telephone, to speak with his daughter. To call up someone who had once been Francis's little girl and explain to her that her father, once strong and able, was at the end of his battle with cancer, that we were stopping his anti-cancer drugs and would increase his pain meds as needed, just about tore me apart. The only reason I did not join her in openly weeping was because Francis was doing his best to console her and let her know it was all OK, there was no reason to cry. An observer could easily have been confused as to who was the dying patient in the situation. I must admit that Francis was not the same in the days after this discussion with his daughter. I think when he first came in he was in denial about what was going on. He talked about getting back to Omaha and doing things with his grandchildren. It was only after our family meeting that he realized he would return to Omaha, but only for his funeral. He had come to Grand Island to die.

I was careful to wrap up clinic quickly my last day at the VA, not only so I could make it back to Lincoln in time for a late supper with my family, but because I could not leave without saying goodbye to Francis. He thanked me for all the time I had spent visiting with him and taking care of a wound that had developed on his backside during his stay. I told him I would not be seeing him from that point on, and that Julie, who had supervised me and who had set up the family meeting, would be his primary provider for the rest of his stay. I doubt if Francis would have cared if I had left that day without saying goodbye. Part of me believes that he knew; I visited one last time not so he would feel better about me leaving, but so that I could feel better about it.

Psychology
Lincoln, Nebraska

I **was not looking forward to** my next rotation. Due to the difficult subject matter, the severity of the cases, or the fact that I might see some part of myself in the patients, psychology was not my cup of tea. Worse yet was that I was to serve my time at the Community Mental Health center in Lincoln. This tax-dollar-funded mental health center was not built to serve the housewife suffering from postpartum depression. The patients here dwelled at the bottom of society, likely because of their mental illness. Since the center was funded by state dollars, it turned away no one, whereas other psych practices in town could, as long as the patient was "stable." This also meant that when a suicide attempt came into the ED of the hospital next door, we were in charge of the intake interview.

The worst part without doubt was that my preceptor, Dr. Sandoval, asked me the first day I met him if I was going to work in psych after graduating. I should have lied, but instead I confessed, "No, I'm probably going to go into surgery of some sort, possibly ortho."

"Oh, well, then I won't waste your time with too many of the details." In essence, my two weeks were spent watching while they conducted their interviews during clinic visits and seeing an occasional suicide attempt at the ED next door, or (if I was lucky) taking a "long lunch" which stemmed from noon to "see you tomorrow."

Looking back now, I am not all that surprised at this attitude, having read *I'm Dancing as Fast as I Can* (Barbara Gordon) and *Voluntary Madness* (Norah Vincent), both written from the perspective of a patient in psychiatric care (both inpatient and outpatient). I am not here to sell her books, but I do highly recommend *Voluntary Madness* due to the fact that Ms. Vincent, who truly is a mental illness patient, voluntarily commits herself to three different facilities and gives a truthful account of her experiences. From this I certainly learned that the more you pay for psychiatric care, the more benefit you will receive and the more one-on-one time you will be given. Ms. Vincent benefited the least from her state-run facility, which was akin to the facility at which I found myself at the time. Looking back, I can see how the apathy of the patients had affected my preceptor and made him apathetic. The patients' resistance to change had led to lack of effort by the physician to help the patients change. I vowed I would never let myself become apathetic, and, thus far, I have thankfully been successful.

The physician preceptor had brushed me aside, so I had to do my best to gain as much knowledge and experience as possible from the nurse practitioner who worked alongside him. Of course, I also had to take advantage of my early dismissals to study for my next quarterly meeting. These testing/discussion sessions occurred about every third rotation, took place on campus, and included a test on every mandatory rotation we had completed since the last one. After the OB/GYN debacle I was looking forward to a successful quarterly meeting, and I was going to use being brushed aside to my advantage.

On my first day in the outpatient clinic, after Dr. Sandoval had established that I was not going into psych, he had me observe him with his first patient of the day, Edgar. Dr. Sandoval introduced me as a student, and Edgar was more than happy to have me there. "Nice to meet you. Teehee."

I was quick to learn that after just about everything Edgar said came an odd smile and that nervous laugh. I had never seen this before in my life. Talk about getting thrown into psych headfirst. I listened as Dr. Sandoval and Edgar talked about day-to-day goings on, which I suppose should have been a clue to the diagnosis, but I had honestly never seen anything like it, nor read about it, and was a bit taken aback.

"Have you been able to gain employment in the community, Edgar?"

"Well, I have called a few places needing part-time help, mostly restaurants, but no job yet. Teehee."

"I see. You are still living with your mother then. You have not been able to afford an apartment of your own without employment, I am guessing."

"Yeah, I still live with mom in the basement. Teehee." After establishing that virtually nothing had changed since the last visit, Dr. Sandoval told Edgar to keep his head up, keep taking his meds, and if any of his previous symptoms return he should go to the hospital ED so he could be quickly attended to. That was the information I bit on, because I was truly stumped as to what was going on inside Edgar's head.

"So, Sean, what mental illness does Edgar have?"

"I would say depression. His nervous laugh is not really leading me to think anxiety, and so I will have to go with bipolar disorder."

Dr. Sandoval was kind enough to pause and consider that answer, making it look like it was halfway intelligent. I appreciated that, because when he told me the real answer I saw just how far off target I was. "Edgar suffers from schizophrenia. He has never really been sad, but sometimes that is the problem. You would think a young man so advanced in life, who is not a teenager, not a twenty-something like you, would strive to move out of his mother's basement, to gain a job, that this failure would sadden him. But his affect is so muted, and that laugh, a common symptom of schizophrenia by the way, makes him seem giddy. From that I can see bipolar, but, no, he is schizophrenic." It wasn't even a rare disorder I had never heard of, one with an abbreviated name longer than some other diagnoses, like schizoaffective disorder, bipolar subtype. It had to be simple schizophrenia. This was going to be a tough test to prepare for in only two weeks.

I spent most days either with the aforementioned physician preceptor or his APRN, Susan. Susan was more driven, but she also had the benefit of her population of patients being more stable than Dr. Sandoval's. Most of her patients had been inpatients already and had gotten over the worst aspect of their mental illness and had treatment plans in place. Also of benefit to her was her background. In my opinion, nurse practitioners are well suited for psychiatric medicine because of their nursing background, which focuses on and emphasizes the patient's needs, wants, and overall care. Not that this is lacking in the PA model, but it is a wonderful aspect of the APRN model—well suited for listening and helping all patients, but greatly suited for psychiatric patients. Susan was a wonderful role model for how psychiatric medicine can be.

Interestingly enough, having struck out with my first patient with Dr. Sandoval, the first patient I saw in outpatient clinic with Susan really did have depression with anxiety. Margaret walked in, followed by Susan, and after introductions were made the visit began. Margaret seemed to be in very good spirits, especially considering her diagnosis. She was nothing like the woman on paper in her chart, which I reviewed during the visit while listening to updates on her condition. Her ED note[3] read,

> Middle-aged female presents this evening tearful and with chief complaint of unbearable depression. Denies suicidal ideation, but states "I cannot go on like this anymore." Depression screening shows moderate to severe depression with underlying anxiety but without suspicion for harm to self or others. At discharge patient hand carries script for SSRI antidepressant, benzodiazepine anxiety relief and recommendation to enroll in outpatient group therapy at local psych clinic.

---

3   Abbreviated to leave out identifying details

Margaret had completed group therapy, to great benefit, and had titrated up to an adequate dosage of her SSRI, and had been weaned off of her benzos. "I feel a million times better now, like the person I was before was just a shell of a woman and now I am full again. Full of potential for happiness."

Susan sat scanning the documentation from previous visits, looking for issues that might still be lingering. "So last time we spoke you had still had a few issues with anxiety, specifically with work stressors. Tell me how that is going."

Margaret's face fell slightly. "Well, yeah, that is still there, but what do you expect? You can't expect perfection when it comes to your boss and co-workers. I am just trying to focus on me, you know? I can't change them, I can only change the way they affect me."

Susan nodded in agreement. "But you are doing OK on just the one medication, now that we have you off the other?"

"Yeah I think so. I know you can't be on those pills forever. We talked in group about how they are a Band-Aid while the other drug builds up and I learn how to work through life. I feel better overall."

I was pleased to see Margaret doing so well; everyone in medicine strives for success, and it is not always so forthcoming. In fact, it could easily be argued that short of fighting cancer, there is no other more difficult fight in medicine than fighting off mental illness. I was certainly delighted to see this level of success come out of group therapy. Group was where I spent three days of my psych rotation—Tuesdays and Thursdays— and it was not so easy to see success on the horizon of these patients.

I really did think I would enjoy group therapy. I am a talker. Anyone who knows me knows I love to talk. I have an Irish background, and likely it is just a touch of the blarney. Group is supposed to be talking and listening and interacting, but it is not. There are people like Margaret who live in the community—not a threat to themselves or others—and then there are the people who live "upstairs" on the second floor of the clinic who don't need "inpatient-inpatient" care, but still desire a structured safe community. (This in contrast to true inpatient over at the hospital for the people who don't have much say, desperately need to be admitted, and sometimes are forced by law to stay a period of time.) Some of the people upstairs were deemed too dangerous to be allowed out on the street, yet not dangerous enough for admission to the hospital, so upstairs they lived under the same level of security as on a normal hospital floor. The rest of the group was out in the world trying to function the best they could, but doing poorly enough that they needed more than the occasional discussion in the office. Some of these people were back for their second, third, or even fourth round of group therapy, because discussions one-on-one with a therapist had proven to be not enough for them.

Each day was split into two sessions: morning and afternoon. The morning was mostly taken up with exercises on paper to open up discussion on various topics deemed important to recovery and improvement for depressive disorders, which was the greatest complaint of most of the participants. Participation was not mandatory, though it was certainly encouraged. The afternoon was slightly more in depth because each individual participated (whether they wanted to or not). As such, the discussions delved deeper into the issues that had led the patient to their current state of mind. As interesting as that may sound, to a future ortho PA right after lunch, these were the longest afternoons of my entire life.

The third and final part of my rotation was rounding on the inpatient floor of the adjacent hospital. It was, surprisingly, the least enjoyable aspect of my psych rotation. This was not because these were the truly ill (mostly the suicide attempts kept for safe keeping), or that it was inpatient medicine (I love inpatient medicine), but because this same floor was the one my father was transferred to seven years prior after his nervous breakdown. I only visited the ward once, since I spent most of my time on the adolescent psych ward (perhaps because depressed, suicidal teenage girls were more prevalent than depressed, suicidal middle-aged men) but it brought back a few too many memories. I considered myself lucky to be a visitor again and still not a resident, and yet it didn't feel much different from the last time. The individual I visited was not depressed like my father had been; he was a young schizophrenic patient named Adam. My preceptor thought it best that I learn about the disease since it is very prevalent in society, yet not all that greatly understood (as demonstrated by my first encounter). Even now I find it difficult to fully understand. Adam told me he hated the voices in his head and didn't want to do what they said. Yet none of his medications was able to quiet them enough that he could hold a job or even live alone in his apartment.

Up to our visit, and immediately thereafter, he had earphones in his ears because the music drowned out the voices telling him to harm himself. "They are always there, and I can't quiet them. Not that I listen to them, but it is distracting. Imagine trying to work or draw or read and there is someone sitting across the table from you talking incessantly. Impossible right? Now add that the person talking to you wants you to hurt yourself or drown your cat or burn the house down *and* put them inside your head, so you can't just leave that room or that building or go anywhere because that voice lives inside you and it hates you."

This analysis pretty much blew me away, but not as much as the answer to my follow-up question. "Is the voice there now? What is it saying?"

"It wants me to kill you, but don't worry; I won't." As comforting as that was to hear, it was disturbing nonetheless. I not only wanted to leave because there was a voice in Adam's head telling him to kill me, but I wanted to leave so that Adam could put his earphones back on. He didn't want to hear that voice any more than I wanted to hear that the voice wanted me dead. I also got the feeling that Adam knew he had been selected for me to see due to how interesting his illness was, and this made him feel like he was on display. If anything, from this rotation I did learn that the stereotypical and stigmatized schizophrenic is not what the disease truly is. It may be true that the homeless person wandering down the street talking to himself is suffering from the disease, and fighting (or just talking to) the voice in his head. Or he might be super lonely, might be thinking out loud—hell, I have done it by accident myself when alone in my house, and I am free of the disease. In fact, schizophrenia is a myriad other symptoms, and is much deeper than that. It is not just hearing voices; it is delusions, impaired speech and mood, and change in personality. It leads to great hardship for patients affected by it due to diminished social skills, inability to care for themselves, and disruption of their day-to-day lives. As much as I disliked my psych rotation, I can at least say I learned much about this disorder.

I was crafty when I set up my psych rotation and am not going to say that I expected anything wonderful from it. I knew it was not my cup of tea, so I did take the opportunity to shorten my suffering a little bit. In order to allow the students to sit for their tests at the quarterly meetings, my PA program cuts short the rotation prior to the testing session by two days, so that tests may be administered on Thursday and graded by Friday for review. I very craftily set up my rotation schedule so that psych fell before a testing session; I believe many of my classmates did as well.

Family Practice II
McCook, Nebraska

Even better than escaping the psych ward (without being ensnared in a catch-22 situation where psychiatry drives you crazy or you are crazy for enjoying it) was that my next rotation was at the family practice clinic in my home town of McCook, Nebraska, with my own family doctor and somewhat hero, Dr. Weston (or Dr. W if you are super close to her and get cleared for informal exchanges—I did not dare) and my other medicine hero, Will the PA. Will did try to talk me into becoming an APRN since they have even more autonomy than PAs (but not in the Midwest where the rules restrict them to almost the same level of freedom), but how can you not look up to a ripped, Hummer-driving, athletic guy with great hair who is adored by patients?

I fell in love with science as a child; I fell in love with biology in junior high; and thanks to my mother's nursing magazines lying around the house, I fell in love with medicine in high school. Yet after all that was said and done, if I was going into medicine the ultimate goal was to be Will and to work with Dr. Weston. Furthermore, there was the fact that more than a few employees at the clinic were looking forward to me graduating PA school and coming back to McCook to work there. My mother is the employee health/infection control nurse at the hospital, and my father was a floor nurse there before taking a travel job with another clinic. You could say McCook Community Hospital/Clinic runs through my veins, and the Conroys run through the veins of the hospital.

The only strange thing was seeing patients. If one were to draw the hierarchy of medicine I don't know where PA/Medical/Nursing/anything students fall (I know we outrank the pink ladies because, although none of us get paid, students are HIPAA certified). I do know that as a student when you are in the middle of a procedure on a patient, you take the role of provider (even though you are well supervised by a real one). As such, when a need for assistance arises you may make a request for a nurse to gather supplies, offer an extra hand, just like a certified provider would. However, these nurses (Karen could probably remember almost getting popped in the nose by young Sean when she gave him his pre-kindergarten shots) had seen me grow from a snot-nosed kinder-gartener to a white-coat-wearing PA student. I cannot imagine they relished taking direction from someone they had virtually helped raise.

Walking into this rotation was different from each of the previous because I was not nervous about meeting the nurses and doctors. I knew almost all of them and supposed they were looking forward to having me around almost as much as I was looking forward to being there. Despite being located in a town of only about eight thousand people, this was the first clinic in which I had worked that there were tablet-computers you could carry from room to room in order to look up labs, read the dictation from prior visits, and document in the electronic medical record (EMR) while talking to the patient.

This experience helped me hit the ground running when I landed my first job in Kansas City and was handed a tablet-PC to document patient encoun-ters. This was also the first rotation where I called in my own prescriptions for patients without anyone hovering over me to make sure I did not make a mistake. (Mistakes weren't possible since I had Epocrates, a mobile app, open so I could read the dosage directly to the pharmacist—all I had to do was know how to multiply and get the number of pills correct.) For the first time I was given my own office in an empty space next to the billing office; I would be spending six weeks here and might as well settle in. The only downside was this was just before Christmas, and so I had only about five months before gradu-ation. This meant I had to spend a fair amount of every lunch time returning calls to recruiters, to clinic managers either setting up on-site interviews for what little time I had available in January to travel, or actually participating in phone interviews. It was about this time that I started to suspect that all the good jobs go to PAs with experience, and any job willing to hire a new grad was doing so because it had been passed over by enough PAs with experience that the hiring manager had become desperate. Every job that sounded great, or where I fell in love with the prospect of having that job during the interview, was "looking for someone with more experience." I think I went on at least two dozen job interviews before I finally received two job offers less than twen-ty-four hours apart at the twenty-fourth hour in late April.

I tried to spend as much time as possible with Dr. Weston, but to truly get experience I had to spend days with the other doctors and the PAs, including Will. It was with Will that I was introduced to the sweet, older ladies who, regardless of your title and education, insist on calling you Dr. {insert last name here}. I had numerous exchanges similar to those Will had all day. "Hello, Dr. Conroy"

"Hello. You can just call me Sean."

"OK, Dr. Sean it is." This almost makes me a little proud, to have had the same problem as the PA I looked up to, because this isn't so much a mistake or lack of information as much as it is respect and appreciation for PAs and the knowledge they possess and the care they provide. I quote one of my more recent patients, "I know what you are, but you work just as hard to get here, and I'm going to call you *doctor*!"

Will has one of the best bedside manners I have ever seen in my life. The first patient we saw together was cordial with me but ecstatic to see Will. I gathered all of her information and a list of the topics she hoped to discuss that day. Will got a bear hug and a fist full of pictures of her grandkids. Even the older gentlemen greeted him with a firm handshake and a belly laugh. The mothers of sick children seemed to breathe a sigh of relief (even after my initial assessment) when Will entered the room. I guess the cape was invisible.

It was on this rotation that I worked with my first Doctor of Osteopathic medicine, Dr. Murphy. Looking back, I am glad that I was able to because my first supervising physician after graduating was a DO. Medical Doctors (MDs) are trained much like PAs are; DOs learn the same things but also learn about therapeutic manipulation—the osteopathic aspect of medicine (osteo referring to bones). They are the perfect meld of doctor and chiropractor inasmuch as they can tweak you but also treat your sinus infection with antibiotics. Before this rotation I was not sure how DOs compared to MDs, but I finished this rotation better informed about these members of the healthcare team.

We saw numerous typical patients: hypertension, diabetes, snotty baby, etc. On top of this, we saw a few patients who had tweaked their backs or had pain in their necks from being hunched over computers all day. The dog groomer who came in for back pain one day provided a type of visit I had never before experienced. Misty was the wife of one of my co-workers from high school, and so was excited to see me and catch up.

However, the conversation was a bit staccato as Dr. Murphy performed her adjustment. "So Sean—" *harrumph* "—how have things been?"

"Oh pretty good. School has been keeping me busy."

"I can imagine. I bet—" *oof* "—PA school is pretty intense." After a few turns, pulls, and pops, Misty was off to pick up her kids from daycare and tell her husband all about running into me at the clinic.

I was able to meet a new graduate PA on this rotation, and to see what it was like to be on your own for the first time. Katherine was very intelligent, but like any new grad was still a bit timid in some aspects of practicing medicine and wanted to consult her supervising physician more than an experienced PA would. Unfortunately, she was under the most foreboding and, dare I say, condescending physician in the practice. (I specifically requested that I not spend any time with him, if at all possible. Luckily, there were so many providers at this clinic that it was possible.) I did have to watch her suffer under his scrutiny when I was with Will and Dr. Murphy, though. (Dr. Murphy was not her supervising physician. I won't even give her doctor a pseudonym or any more space than necessary.) Katherine could do no right. He acted more like a preceptor than any preceptor I had had up to that point, even though he was speaking with a colleague. I get that he wanted her to think things through, but he was way more than just arrogant; he was a special kind of jerk. I began praying that day that whomever I worked under while practicing medicine would be nothing like her supervising physician. Thus far, I have been fairly lucky, only suffering mild abuse in my first position and none since—at least not at the hands of physicians. I have also been graced with the collegial presence of excellent nurses my whole career, and that is probably more important that one's supervising physician anyway. It was probably fortunate that I did not gain employment at McCook Clinic. This meant I neither had this pompous physician overseeing me nor a clinic nurse who had cared for me as I grew in the community.

Not only had I been cared for as an obnoxious child by some of the nurses in the clinic, but some of the patients I saw in clinic were also all too familiar with a much younger version of me. In fact, before I was escorted to the back on my first day, the mother of my first girlfriend (well, she wore my baseball cap during recess in sixth grade) walked up to me and said, "Oh, Sean, we are all so proud of you becoming a doctor!"

"Thank you, but technically I am going to be a PA."

"That's the same thing. You guys work just as hard to get where you are going. We are just *so proud*!" Of course, emotions other than pride likely exist when you are sitting on the exam table waiting to disclose an embarrassing detail about your body and in walks Sean whom you baby sat. Most patients were understanding.

It helped that Lisa, the nurse I worked with under Dr. Weston, would ask, "Do you know Sean Conroy? He is a PA student with us today, and, if it is OK he will get things rolling." At least then they had fair warning.

There were a few patients who didn't care one bit that they had known me as a child and oddly looked forward to my opinion on their health. Case in point: One day during my lunch break I ran down to the gas station that my sister used to manage. The girl behind me in line asked if I was Steph's brother, which I confirmed, as well as the fact that I was at the clinic doing a family practice rotation. "Great I have an appointment there later on today. Maybe I will see you." I did see her later on that day for mastitis. (She had just had a child and was breastfeeding him and her breast had become infected.) She had no problem disrobing for her friend's brother, whom she had met at the gas station that day, because Steph had told her I was a smart guy.

Another memorable patient around my age was a girl from my high school class (a member of the student council I served on) who was pregnant and, due to elevated blood pressure, was being seen weekly in clinic to make sure she and the baby were doing well. The first visit was awkward, especially with the fear looming of a possible pelvic exam, but once she realized that this was unlikely and that should it be necessary she was free to request someone else to do it she relaxed, and each week she became accustomed to me caring for her.

Strangely, I had more trouble keeping the patients at ease the closer they were to my parents' age. One female patient cowered behind her purse upon seeing me, despite the fact that she was just there to get her cholesterol medication refilled and was welcome to, if not encouraged to, keep all her clothes on during the visit. Completing the cohort of patients were the older ones who either didn't know me since I was too young to be familiar, or, if they did know me, they had been in worse situations in life and had no problems with me seeing them in the clinic.

One morning while I was working with Dr. Weston, my great-uncle on my father's side had a terrible nosebleed—but not so bad that he needed the emergency room—and presented to the clinic. I was more than happy to see him; given his situation, he was less than happy to see anyone.

"I don't care who you send in just get this damn nosebleed to stop!" I heard him holler at the nurse as I waited outside the door. There are various methods of treating an errant nosebleed, and being the good student I am I explained each to him, with pros and cons, and decided we would place a nasal tampon which he would leave in for twenty-four hours and then come back for removal the next day. "Great! Whatever! Just do it!" Like a good patient he returned the next day in much better spirits and we were able to make small talk and catch up a bit.

During this rotation, I placed my first urinary catheter to collect a specimen on a nursing home resident who was the mother of the grocery manager I had worked under all through high school. Neither the patient nor her son was bothered that a student placed her urinary catheter. Yet it was a bit odd that her son, the grocery store manager, wanted to hear all about my life while I placed a tube into his mother's urethra. Whether a nursing home patient or son in his sixties, the older they were, the less they cared.

I am hesitant to go into detail about too many specific patients in this chapter, but will certainly discuss another aspect of family medicine I became aware of during this rotation: drug representatives. Virtually not a day went by the entire six weeks I was there that a representative from one drug company (sometimes two) did not appear with food, snacks, lunch, pens, or other trinkets, and, of course, the latest greatest research that showed their drug was the best on the market for the disease it treated.

I thought I could get off lucky, snag some free food and swag, and then duck back out. "I'm just a student. I don't have prescribing privileges."

"No matter, let me tell you about my wonder drug!" I came to find out that PA students are like the children of religious zealots and Cornhusker fans: indoctrinate them young and win them over for life. The drug reps figured if they could win me over at the start of my career they could glean years of me loyally prescribing their drug—name brand only if they were really good. Of course, to be a PA student you are likely intelligent enough to see right through this ploy, but that did not stop me from paying the price of listening to a biased medical lecture from a salesman in order to get a free doughnut. It was shortly after this that the government clamped down on drug reps and barred them from giving out physical goods such as pens, stethoscope tags, etc. Food, drug samples, and literature were all that were allowed. This was in hopes of decreasing the influence the drug reps have on providers; however, I can tell you personally the drug companies are the ones who benefited. Providers will come listen to you talk for free food just as much as free food and a pen, and no, we aren't necessarily buying your spiel. Not to say I never used the drugs the reps told me about, but if I did it is because I had done my homework, and the unbiased studies supported its use.

I still didn't have a job locked down but had plenty of interviews on my calendar, and had learned a great deal from a great number of wonderful medical professionals. Having replenished my supply of pens and notepads, and having eaten as many free sandwiches as one person can possibly eat, it was time for me to depart McCook and my last true general medicine rotation. From here on out it was specialties only, starting with cardiology.

Cardiology
Location Changed

I really thought I was going to enjoy my cardiology rotation. Every specialty will tell you why theirs is the most important. Neurology because without a brain to send signals along nerves how can the body work? Pulmonology because the body cannot function without oxygen. Cardiology because without a pump to push that oxygen to the lungs and brain nothing gets done. That is actually a pretty strong argument. However, this rotation made me so miserable I am going pretend it took place in Lexington, Kentucky, at Carolina Cardiology to protect the guilty. This was the rotation that ruined Nurse Practitioners for me until my first job where I worked with two young APRNs fresh out of school who had not yet formed vendettas against PAs. This rotation made me quiver in fear around older APRNs and duck behind nurses' stations until they had passed. It wasn't until 2012, and my first family practice job, that a wonderful experienced APRN named Lynetta was able to right the ship and bring me back around.

I remember it being dark out when I arrived for my first day, which was to be spent in surgery in the hospital connected to the outpatient cardiac center. Perhaps I should have felt the black cloud over me from day one. I found my PA preceptor, Bill, who escorted me to the men's changing room and warned me about Dr. Gupta. "He is one of the best cardiologists in the country. Probably too good. You have heard of Louisville Cardiology, haven't you? Well, Dr. Gupta actually helped start this practice, left us for Louisville due to politics, ran into politics there, decided our issues were better, and came back. The thing is his patients followed him there and back. He is that good, but he knows it."

Wow, I thought to myself, this is going to be an interesting rotation. But as long as I do what I am told, follow instructions, and follow the mid-level's lead I felt I should be fine. Though it is usually a reason to worry when the first thing you learn on your rotation after the men's room door code is how much the surgeon loves himself. We scrubbed into surgery, which was to be a bypass to treat a blockage that had caused a heart attack, and got down to business under the supervision of Dr. Gupta. My role was again retractor master until the rib spreader had separated the sternum and exposed the beating heart, and then a brace was put into place holding the surgical site open. From there on out, I was an awestruck observer.

Early in the procedure Dr. Gupta asked me if I had ever held a beating human heart in my hand. Of course, I had not. "Then this is a golden opportunity for you." He gently guided my hand behind the patient's heart. It felt warm and slick as it pulsated rhythmically in my hand. This proved to be the highlight of my stint in cardiology.

The patient was placed on cardiopulmonary bypass while a machine operated by a clinical perfusionist took over the roles of the heart and lungs oxygenating blood and pumping it back into the patient while Dr. Gupta sewed a vessel to bypass the blockage that had led to the ischemic event. I don't recall the procedure being all that long, perhaps because I was in awe, but there was a period when time seemed to stop near the end. After successfully grafting the bypass onto the occluded artery of the heart it was time for the heart to take over pumping blood to the body, and for the patient to come off of the bypass machine. Dr. Gupta asked for the cardiac paddles, which would shock the heart back into its normal rhythm. "Everybody clear!" Zap. On the wall at the head of the bed was the largest TV I had seen up to that point, and on it was the EKG strip corresponding to our patient's heart rate. In TV shows they like to show a patient going flat line. No one goes flat line in real life; instead, they go into an erratic rhythm that looks like a child scribbling, the scribbles determined by the electrical current of the failing heart. However, when the heart is artificially stopped and placed on bypass, you do see an almost straight line on the EKG. This line persisted after the first shock.

"Nothing, OK, clear again . . . zap . . . stay clear . . . zap . . . almost." After eight shocks we finally got a good scribble, but of course that was not what we were going for.

Dr. Gupta watched the scribbles intently. "Ventricular fibrillation . . . zap . . . V-fib . . . zap."

This entire cascade of events probably lasted all of two minutes, but it felt like an eternity. I was certain we weren't going to get the heart started, the wife and kids, the grandkids . . . oh I do not want to hear this discussion, when on the eleventh attempt the heart fluttered into a normal sinus rhythm.

"Excellent, Bill, sternum wire please." Dr. Gupta took the thick wire used to close the sternum and began closing the rib cage around the beating heart. Once it was placed and the closure was down to the soft tissue of the skin, Dr. Gupta handed off to Bill, and Bill finished closing the case, teaching me his favorite closure method.

My first two weeks of this rotation were actually fairly enjoyable, because Bill took the time to teach me. Bill and I scrubbed into cases which took all morning and, of course, a few emergency ones in the afternoon. For the most part, afternoons were spent in the "Cath lab," where small blockages and simpler cases were fixed via an angiocatheter inserted into a vein in the leg and then passed up into the heart where a small balloon (angioplasty is the name of the procedure) was inflated, widening the occluded area. These patients are sick, don't get me wrong, but have enough flow past the area of interest that they typically have to wait until after lunch and are scheduled back to back. This was less interesting than open-heart surgery, but still very interesting as I sat behind a desk with a tall glass divider watching Dr. Gupta open arteries clogged by cholesterol plaques.

Likely the most interesting case of the entire rotation was a gentleman younger than me. Dr. Gupta, while he specialized in cardiac illness, is actually a cardiothoracic surgeon, meaning he can perform surgeries related to the heart but also those related to the cavity within which the heart resides. This young man had presented to his primary care provider with cool fingers and a slight weakness in his left arm. After an extensive workup, including a CT scan, it was determined that a previous left clavicle (collarbone) fracture had healed in so thick there was a compression of the vessels and nerves running to the left arm between the healed fracture and the first rib on that side. Conservative measures had failed to alleviate his symptoms so it was decided to take the young man to the operating room and free up the compressed soft structures by removing the compressing fracture callus of the clavicle, and, just for good measure, placing a notch in the first rib. I found this case to be the most interesting due to the rarity of the condition and the rarity of needing surgical intervention to treat it. There are numerous conditions that can lead to thoracic outlet syndrome, but typically surgery is avoided if at all possible, so to find myself participating in such a procedure was an excellent experience. It was certainly different from the procedures I had seen before it and the ones I saw after it on my cardiology rotation; we never even saw the heart as the surgical field was superior and lateral from the center of the chest. The procedure was simple; I imagined an orthopedic surgeon performing it just as easily with a hand-held burr used during shoulder surgeries. I would say that patient in, patient back to recovery, the case probably took less than an hour, but having Dr. Gupta show me everything involved, having him discuss the anatomy of a rare condition was certainly worth scrubbing in for.

After two weeks of surgery it was time for me to move across the parking lot to the outpatient clinic on the first floor and upstairs to cardiac step-down. The inpatients upstairs in the hospital were either waiting for their surgery or were recovering from it. The outpatients in clinic had already had surgery, or a few rare ones had not yet gotten bad enough for surgery but were complicated enough that a specialist was necessary to manage their condition. This included pediatric patients born with cardiac anomalies or adults who had once been pediatric cardiology patients and, thanks to interventions, had survived to adulthood and presented on occasion just to verify they were still doing well.

Before I left, Bill warned me that the APRNs who were taking over as my preceptors were to be approached cautiously. "They are catty, they are perfectionists, and, truthfully, they are bitches, if I may be so forward and vulgar. Keep your head down and just survive these next two weeks. On Tuesday and Thursday afternoons I work over in the interrogation room[4], I will see to it that you are there with me those four days, but the other six . . . Just keep your head down. Trust me, they don't like PAs. Oh, and by the way, I will do your mid-rotation evaluation later on today. Don't worry; you did fine." My biggest fear was that these "catty" APRNs were to do my final and most important evaluation. It was time to go into suck-up mode.

The following Monday I began what can only be described as the most terrible two weeks of my life. Bill didn't have an office; he had a locker outside the surgical area and he had a desk in the interrogation room where he kept pictures of his daughters. This desk became an oasis away from the nurse practitioners. I met Lucy in the office she shared with Fern that first day and introduced myself as her PA preceptee. Why the class ahead of me warned me about Dr. Phillips in York, but not about these two is beyond me.

"Great, let's get to rounds." She walked out the door as I set my bag down. I grabbed my PDA with all my medical software and a pen and paper in case I needed to make notes, and scrambled to catch up. I caught up as the elevator doors opened, and we stepped in to ride up to the second floor where the inpatients were. I wondered if she would have waited for me. I had never been to the second floor of the hospital, but she did not know that or seem to care. She stepped out and took a hard left to the nurses' station.

"The charts are behind the counter. Grab the charts for 202, 208, and 212. You can see those. Meet me back here after." She didn't introduce me to the nurses, didn't open a chart to show me how it was organized, and didn't tell me exactly what it was she wanted to know about each patient. Now, don't get me wrong; a student should know their way around a medical interview and

---

4   Not nearly as interesting as you might think. Pacemakers have batteries and very small computers inside them that monitor not only battery charge, but also defibrillations and other activity. A magnet is placed over the pacer/defibrillator to turn it off, and then the information can be downloaded. You "interrogate" the device.

physical exam, should be able to scratch out a quick SOAP note[5]. This was, however, a specialty and it would have been nice to know precisely what it was this service focused on. If I had come back with, "the patient has a runny nose," would it have been helpful? A little guidance would have been appreciated.

I found my way into the chart for room 202, a seventy-six-year-old female who had been downstairs in the cath lab the day before, and had a surgical note describing the procedure and the vessel that had been opened. She was in good spirits and feeling well that day. She was ready to go home, she said. I explained that I was just a student, but that I would talk to the APRN about it. Luckily, I had seen an angioplasty before and I read the operative report to know where the incision was on her right thigh. I pulled her sheets out of the way, put on gloves, and peeled back the bandage. The surgical site was moist, but did not appear infected. I placed the bandage back down. I continued with a brief physical exam: heart, lungs, abdomen, checked her ankles for swelling, and found her to be doing as well as she had claimed. I informed her I would let Lucy know, and we would be back shortly with a firm plan for her care.

I proceeded to the nurses' station, swapped out 202 for 208 and began reading about that gentleman. A fifty-six-year-old male who had a bypass the previous week, which I had actually scrubbed in on. I reviewed the operative note to recall the specifics, and checked his post-operative labs. They all looked reasonable: specifically, no anemia. I read the previous rounding notes and gained some insight as to what was expected on rounds.

I had done fairly well on the first patient, jotted down some labs I might want for her on my scratch paper, and headed into 208. "Good morning. How are you today? You probably don't remember me, but when Dr. Gupta performed your bypass, I assisted his assistant."

"You don't say. So you are pretty low on the totem pole then, assistant to the assistant. Does that pay well?"

"Well, actually I pay for the privilege. I am a PA student."

"Hell of a note!" he laughed, and instantly grimaced in pain from having done so. "Oh boy, you can't crack any more jokes. I might die laughing!"

I agreed it would be strictly business from there on out. I peeled his gown open and, after donning gloves, investigated his surgical site, which was healing nicely. I gave him the same exam as 202 and, finding him doing well, informed him I would discuss his care with Lucy, the APRN, and we would return with the game plan.

---

5   Subjective, Objective, Assessment, Plan. How does the patient feel, how is the patient medically, what findings came out of the visit, and what are you going to do based on that?

Back to the nurses' station for my last chart: 212. Another angio patient, this one a sixty-one-year-old male. He looked worn out, and let me know right way. "I feel like crap!"

I reviewed his chart and noted he had a slightly elevated white blood cell count. "Looks like you might have an infection going on somewhere inside you. Tell me more about feeling like crap."

"I just feel worn out. I can't even get up to go pee. Run over by a bus describes it nicely."

I noticed the urinary catheter collection bag hanging at the end of his bed. Inside was yellow, but cloudy urine. "Well, first place to look would probably be sending some urine to the lab to see if your infection is in your bladder."

I donned gloves to investigate his surgical site, right upper thigh. Under the bandage was a clean, healing wound. "This looks good. That would be the only other likely source of infection after surgery. Let me listen to you here."

I placed the stethoscope against his chest. His revascularized heart was beating inside his chest, his lungs sounded clear. Thus, I was fairly certain he had a UTI, and this was the source of his elevated white blood cell count. Being wiped out was both contributory and a result, I surmised. I returned to the nurses' station and settled in behind a computer next to where the charts were kept. A few nurses stopped by and inquired as to whether I was a student and introduced themselves. In the middle of one introduction my preceptor arrived. "Move. That's my chair. What did you find out?"

I quickly vacated the chair and began presenting my patients. "In 202 we have a seventy-six-year-old female, status post angioplasty yesterday. She is in good spirits, says she feels so good she is ready to go home."

"Not gonna happen."

"OK, uh . . . lungs clear, heart regular rate and rhythm, post-operative site is moist but healing well—"

"You took her bandage off?!"

"Well, I lifted it. I had gloves on, just peeked under—"

"Are you *trying* to kill her?!" By now the nurses were all focused on the two of us. Like a shot, Lucy was out of her chair and bolted into 202. I followed. What was I supposed to do?

Lucy shouted over me for a nurse to come in. "Get this dressing off. Clean the surgical site with alcohol and Betadine. Place a new dressing. Right now." The nurse nodded and left to gather supplies. "I cannot believe you put a dirty dressing on my surgical patient." I flushed red with embarrassment.

"I thought he was very nice," interjected the patient.

"Nice won't keep you from getting an infection." Lucy left the room and went back to the nurses' station. Might as well get it over with, I thought.

"Well, I peeked under the dressings of 208 and 212 as well, so . . ."

"The *open heart patient*? Nurse, 208! You! Stay here!" She growled at me, and shot off into 208. This was the first time my entire clinical year when, except for after the death of a patient, I felt tears welling up in my eyes. Still flush from the encounter, too embarrassed to look at the nurses around me, I sat in the chair, and swiveled to face the computer. After a few moments it passed, but I needed some time and space.

"Where is the restroom? Had a few cups of coffee this morning." I faked a small smile best I could.

"You came up in the elevators right? If you go back there, but past them on the left are the restrooms for family that comes to visit. That is the closest one." I proceeded to the restroom and spent a few moments taking deep breaths. I had walked into Lucy's office just before 7 a.m.; it wasn't even 8 yet, and I still had many days before me. After collecting myself, I returned to the nurses' station and waited for Lucy. After what seemed like an eternity, she returned. "Out of my chair."

I moved quickly to the side. She began typing in the computer, logging onto the system. I never even got a chance to present my other two patients. She eventually grabbed their charts, told me I could follow her, and she evaluated them from scratch. She even sent 212's urine to the lab. Looking back, the only thing I can say in my defense is that as an ortho PA we routinely evaluated incisional sites by gently lifting the bandage, and if there was infection, quickly removed the bandage and called the nurses. After our visit, we sent the nurse in to place a new bandage and trusted the nurse to clean the incisional site before doing so. Furthermore, had Lucy told me to not touch the surgical sites I would have gladly complied with her instructions. I feel she was way out of line.

Rounds took all morning. It felt like a week. I was given only a small sampling of the floor to see as I followed Lucy around like a dejected ghost, hardly speaking. Eventually, it was time for lunch, so we proceeded to the break room on the first floor of the hospital. There was a kitchen/cafeteria adjacent for family members to purchase meals and snacks. As a student I was provided meals, and had been the whole rotation thus far. This was the first time I didn't feel like eating on campus. As a starving student, though, you don't really have an option, so I silently ate my sandwich and soup. I could see the looks on the faces of the scrub techs I had worked with the previous two weeks. They seemed to think I was a different person, or I had suffered the death of a loved one. Theirs were looks of pity.

After lunch it was time to go to the outpatient clinic where Lucy and Fern saw patients in the afternoon. I had not yet met Fern, but upon arriving at the clinic we bumped into her. "Fern, this is Sean. He is our *PA* student." She said it the same way a minister would introduce a drug dealer. Fern feigned delight. I appreciated that, but the feeling in the air was that I was far beneath their station. I was assigned a sign-in to the dictation line so that I could see patients and dictate the SOAP notes that resulted from the visit. Though I could tell they didn't want to, it was expected to allow students to see patients, present them to the preceptor, and after the plan was formulated, dictate the note. The schedule was packed, so I would have to write my notes down and dictate them at the end of the day. I didn't mind that; I only hoped I would survive that long.

The afternoon went on without much difficulty. Most patients were post-operative, but a few were just there to discuss their medication and all were doing fine. None that first day had been born with any congenital heart problems. At least the patient load was breaking me in easily. I was able to present the patients to Lucy, didn't have any difficulty answering her follow-up questions, and ended the day almost believing that I had convinced her I had a brain between my ears after all. I entered the dictation room with my stack of notes and began dictating my SOAP notes. Somewhere in the middle of it, Lucy poked her head in. "Tomorrow I will round on all the inpatients. You come over and spend the morning with Fern since we opened up her schedule; in the afternoon you will be with Bill." Then *poof*, she was gone. I had paused my dictation in progress; I hit the keypad to continue, and wrapped up my dictation, which had included a recent echocardiogram.

I am the kind of guy who always has to be doing something, listening to something. Silence unnerves me, but driving home that evening I turned my CD player off and just let the silence envelope me, hoping the calm would treat the storm the day had created. If I am ever diagnosed with post-traumatic stress disorder, my cardiology rotation will be the stressor identified.

The next day, Tuesday, day two (I was glad Bill was going to be my afternoon) I met Fern walking into the lobby of the clinic. "I hear you had some trouble rounding yesterday."

I didn't know how to answer this. I wanted to defend myself, but if I did I would only anger both the APRNs, but to give in felt like I was enabling the abuse. I managed a quick middle line. "I didn't hit the expectations quite right, but I know how to improve in the future." It still felt dirty coming out of my mouth.

"Well you can try again tomorrow. We just wanted to make sure you got some more outpatient experience before heading off to the pacer lab today." My only concern was whether I would have enough time to dictate. I could tell it was either going to be no lunch or getting home late. After the day before I was more than willing to forgo the break room at lunch.

The morning's clinic was about the same as the previous afternoon's. Luckily Fern gave me half an hour to dictate before lunch so I was able to get some lunch in before rushing off to meet Bill on the other side of the clinic in the pacer interrogation clinic. "I see they haven't chewed you up and spit you out yet."

"They dug their claws in. I think they are waiting for me to bleed out. Didn't you see the blood trail when I came in?"

Bill about died laughing. I am glad someone could see the humor in my situation. "Only, what? Eight more days? It's not so long. Sit down. I will give you the run down. This magnet here—we call them donuts—turns the pacer/ defib off and on."

Bill had to use both hands to peel it off of the filing cabinet next to his desk. "Follow me." Bill led me down the hall to one of the exam rooms.

"This is the mobile computer; the girls call it COW, or computer on wheels. With this wand we interrogate the devices."

Throughout the afternoon Bill showed me how to turn the devices off with the magnet, place the wand over the device, and upload the data, which included how often it had defibrillated, what rates it had paced the heart at, including breaks when the heart itself had taken over, and the battery life remaining. A few people were getting toward the end of their pacer life, and were scheduled to talk to Dr. Gupta about the procedure to replace the battery.

The next morning, I was allowed to return to the hospital for rounds, but was not allowed to see patients myself. As I followed Fern from room to room, I felt my cell phone vibrating numerous times in my pocket. Eventually we settled into the nurses' station, and as I watched Fern type in the computer, I could not help but wonder who had called so many times. I excused myself to the restroom, and quickly checked my voicemail. Three different recruiters had called with job opportunities in the space of one hour. I, of course, was pretty excited (little did I know just how common recruiter calls are once your name gets into the world of recruiters) and as much fun as it was watching Fern type, I hoped to be able to call them back. I returned to the nurses' station and meekly asked Fern if I could return the recruiters phone calls. "Sure." She didn't seem to care, so I wandered back towards the restroom/elevator bay and made my calls. I set up one interview and one phone interview, but had to let one possibility slide.

I returned to the nurses' station to find Fern still typing away. "Anything I can do to help?"

"No."

Alrighty then. I took the opportunity to check my email on my PDA.

That afternoon it was back over to the outpatient clinic. First off, I was to spend some time with Dr. Gupta in the echocardiography lab to see echocardiograms, or echos, being performed. Echos give insight into the heart's four chambers, the valves that separate the chambers, and the wall of the heart, letting the doctor know if a problem is arising. The echo sonographer placed the gooed-up wand over the patient's heart, and an upside-down heart appeared on the COW, pulsating on-screen. The blood flowed blue in one direction, stopped quickly, jetted out red, and back and forth. After shifting the wand around to get a clear view, the sonographer saved the file and cleaned up the goo.

Later on, Dr. Gupta reviewed the files, replaying the echo on his computer and scribbling notes to dictate later. Watching the echos reminded me of a lecture from the didactic phase of PA school when a radiologist referred to sonography as, "A nice view of the body, if you stand on your head." It utilizes radio waves bouncing off of the area of interest, but the images are upside down. I found myself wanting to flip the monitor over to look at the heart correctly, but Dr. Gupta seemed to have no trouble. Of course, the best part for me was one less afternoon with Fern and Lucy.

The second week with the APRNs and the final week of cardiology was much like the first. I did my best to keep my head down and survive. A few recruiters called, a few times I escaped to spend time with Bill or Dr. Gupta, and the final day eventually came. "So today we will be evaluating you. How do you think you did?"

Lucy and I were in her office. I was looking forward to leaving.

"I certainly learned a lot. This was a wonderful rotation."

"I didn't ask how we did. I asked how you did. Anyway, I will get it done sometime next week. I want to talk to Fern and Bill about things." I had a knot in my stomach as I walked out that day.

After we took the tests for that quarter I was called into the program director's office. It was the same situation as OB/GYN but worse. One person evaluated me at mid-rotation and gave me wonderful marks; another at the end was less than impressed. The kicker is that my lowest marks were due to the fact that I spent too much time on the phone talking to recruiters (despite having been given permission to do so) and not enough of my free time was spent studying. Most glaring, however (and Lucy actually called to discuss this), was my interpretation of an echo before Dr. Gupta had seen it. He had seen it, he had written his notes, it was in the chart that Lucy had handed me to dictate, and so I did. To quote her, "I wouldn't even feel comfortable interpreting an echo let alone a *student!*"

I tried to explain to the program director that I had assumed the report was final—nowhere did it say preliminary—and I had been asked without any further direction to dictate on the patient. Then, of course, I kissed ass and back peddled. I did request that the director call Bill and have him explain just how much Lucy and Fern disliked PA students. This conversation did occur, and Bill threw me under the bus, saying he had never had any problems with them and was surprised I had done so poorly the second two weeks after having done so well with him. Again, by fortune alone, I received high enough of a score on the written portion to squeak another B and pass the rotation. Apparently one does not need to study feverishly in front of APRNs, as long as one does so at home.

Looking back on it all I guess I should have put on a better front. I should have carried a textbook with me, or at least a packet of notes to study during my downtime. If anything, I should have reviewed EKG interpretation instead of returning recruiter calls once I realized Lucy and Fern were not going to let me round anymore. Perhaps I could have striven for perfection a little harder, heeded Bill's advice a little more. I can forgive Bill, he did warn me about Fern and Lucy. Then when called out in front of the colleagues he warned me about, he of course backpedaled and protected himself; he was stuck with them for years after I escaped. Fern and Lucy I don't think I will ever forgive. I have had a few high school students follow me, and one PA student on a family practice rotation. It is due to these two preceptors on my cardiology rotation that I sit even the high school students down on the first day and asked them "What do you hope to learn during your time here?" After learning their expectations I have always explained my own. There was so little direction, and so much abuse when my misdirected actions did not yield the results expected those last two weeks of my cardiology rotation. I will never forget to use it as a model on how not to precept. Luckily the rotation that followed cardiology not only featured one of my better preceptors, but also cute little kids.

Pediatrics
Lincoln, Nebraska

My first day of pediatrics was a cold February morning in Lincoln, Nebraska, and was right down the street from one of the hospitals I had visited on my orthopedics rotation. I made note of this as pediatrics clinics usually don't have cafeterias, but that hospital has the best doctors' lounge in all of Nebraska (in my opinion). I parked at the far end of the clinic parking lot and found my way into the waiting room where the receptionist greeted me and escorted me back to Dr. Wheeler's office.

Moments later my preceptor arrived and gave me a tour of the office. "Go ahead and pull up a chair on the other side of my desk and make yourself a little office space, then I will show you around. The building is divided in two, myself and my PA, Margaret, work on this side, and the other side is where Dr. Smith and his PA, Abby, work."

The office was very spread out and in fact did have a rather impressive kitchen area if I decided to bring my lunch. "Feel free to put anything in there, snacks, pop, whatever. If drug reps stop by, we always make sure the leftovers get saved. You are always welcome to that." I was ecstatic to get some time with Dr. Wheeler after my abysmal prior rotation.

I was introduced to the nurses, shown where everything was located. "Now this is a pretty busy practice, so I will let you see patients, but since we are taking care of little people, I absolutely have to go in and assess them myself, just for liability. I trust you, so if you can give a good thorough presentation so I can get in and out quickly, things should go great." Telling me his expectations right up front was a great foot to be getting off on. The weather might be frightful, but I could tell this rotation was going to be wonderful. We proceeded back to our shared office space and began the morning discussing the new vaccine schedule (of which I placed a copy in my pocket for reference) before seeing patients in a packed schedule.

It was cold and flu season, so a majority of the kids we saw that day were in for earaches, coughs, and runny noses, but one runny nose and cough stood out against the rest. I began the visit by introducing myself and letting the mother know Dr. Wheeler would be in shortly.

The mother told me about her infant son. "He has had this cough for a few days, but it seems like it is getting worse every day, and now he sounds all wheezy and he has been super fussy and I think he has a fever." I checked and, sure enough, 100.1 axillary, which means he was actually closer to 101. I placed my stethoscope against his chest, complete with pediatric attachment for tiny bodies, and listened. He had a wheeze both inspiratory and expiratory, with a coarse rattle in the background of his breath. His tiny heart raced in the background, but at a normal rate for a person his age. Finally, it was time for nobody's favorite part; peeking at his ears, nose, and throat. He was less than pleased and wrestled with me, but with mom's assistance I was able to see that his ears were fine, he had a runny nose, but nothing terrible, and his throat appeared normal. As the little man wailed his protest I took another listen to his lungs to find out if they had cleared. Sometimes after a child breathes in deeply during a period of crying, maybe even a few coughs, the upper airway will clear and the noises improve; this little man's lung sounds did not. I informed the mother that this did indeed sound like something more impressive than just a cold, and that I should have Dr. Wheeler come in and verify that the little man needed intervention. I exited the room, made my way to "our" office, and began my presentation. I filled in Dr. Wheeler on all the details, and told him that I worried the young patient had bronchiolitis, and was maybe working on a pneumonia.

"Was this patient born at term? Or pre-term?"

I quickly flipped through the chart and found the patient had been born at thirty-four weeks, four days.

"OK, not a true preemie, but still a little early. What do we worry about in preemies?"

I hadn't even thought about this being a case of respiratory synctitial virus (RSV), but quickly realized it definitely could be, and that this little man may require hospitalization.

"Let's grab the pulse ox and check in on him. If it's low we will send him down the street to the hospital for a chest X-ray and RSV swab."

We gathered the additional supplies and returned to the room. Dr. Wheeler listened while I placed the pulse oximeter on the ear of the patient (a nice addition as pediatric patients have really tiny fingers) and it was quickly determined that with an oxygen saturation of 85% and the sounds Dr. Wheeler now heard, that this patient should be sent to the hospital for more tests. As the mother exited to the front of the clinic, Dr. Wheeler picked up the phone and hit speed dial for the hospital blocks away.

"Yeah, this is Wheeler. I am sending a little guy your way, screen for RSV, chest X-ray with stat over-read, even if all that looks good I think we should admit him for O_2/inhaled epi, and steroids." He hung up the receiver and gave me a pearl of wisdom.

"It is easier to break it to the parents that their little guy has to spend some time in the hospital if A: you tell them we need more tests to confirm that it is necessary, kind of put it in their mind, but not firm, and B: if they are already *in* the hospital. It is just down the hall so they don't have to drive there thinking about it."

About an hour later the results were back: bronchiolitis secondary to RSV. The patient was admitted for oxygen supplementation, inhaled epinephrine, and inhaled steroids to open up his lungs while he fought the infection. "It feels good to be right, but you hate to be right about having to admit someone that young." Dr. Wheeler loved his job, but admitted it had its challenges.

On my ortho rotation I had hoped to meet a player or two from a certain local university football team, as the practice, on occasion, consulted with the team physicians, but that did not happen. However, I received an unexpected surprise on my pediatric rotation, since Dr. Wheeler was the pediatrician for the children of more than one coach at the local university of which I am a huge fan, and I was able to see the kids/nieces/nephews of at least one of my idols. It is not quite as exciting getting to see your hero's kids for runny noses when it is his wife who brings them in. I suppose that made it easier to keep my cool during those visits.

More of a bonus, I suppose, was running into one of my classmates from medical technology school, as well as from Chadron State prior to our time at MT school. Caroline brought in her two kids about halfway through my rotation. Both were snotty, but the older child, Larry, was certainly more so. He had been tearful throughout the night and would hardly let anyone touch his right ear. It is never all that easy examining a child, worse if they are sick, and the worst is examining the sick child of a friend. Caroline understood the importance of getting a good look at her sick little guy, and assisted me to peek inside both his ears. The left tympanic membrane was a little red and probably infected; the right one was flaming red with white purulent infection visible behind it. Poor Larry screamed through the entire examination: ears, nose, throat, heart, and lungs. After making my diagnosis of a bilateral ear infection (and checking my own ears to make sure I could still hear), I exited the room to discuss the case with Dr. Wheeler.

I informed him of the cause of the wailing likely heard in every corner of our half of the clinic, and luckily (for Larry, Caroline . . . well all of us), Dr. Wheeler took my word for it and let the poor child escape a second examination.

We prescribed weight-calculated amoxicillin and sent him on his way. The next morning poor Larry was back in our clinic with a dreadful wheeze in his chest and wailed without an invasive physical exam.

"He is still pulling at that right ear, and now he is croupy and wheezy. I just don't know what we are going to do with him," Caroline calmly explained. They say that health care workers are the worst patients, but they are probably the best parents to deal with because, although they won't take themselves to the doctor for things they probably should, they conversely don't freak out unnecessarily when their children are patients. Thus, it was safe to assume that little Larry really was in bad shape or Caroline wouldn't have brought him back so soon. Of course, Murphy's Law dictates that if you see your friend's kids in clinic, they will be the ones who get worse before they get better. I assessed poor Larry again, including his oxygen saturation, which was in the low 90s—low, but not dreadful.

"I bet if we add some nebulized albuterol he will be breathing better. We can give him a treatment here and see if it helps."

"Sounds good to me. Anything to get him feeling better and sleeping better, so I can sleep better . . . and feel better." I could certainly sympathize with that statement, having two young sons of my own. I found Dr. Wheeler and explained my findings, and we had the nurse get him set up with a quick albuterol breathing treatment. About ten minutes later, Larry sounded much better and was in better spirits.

"Do you have a nebulizer at home you can use if we write for the vials? If not, we have some you can rent."

Dr. Wheeler looked at Larry's little sister. "Though with two kids and sharing being caring, you should probably invest in your own."

"Yeah, we actually got one last time, so if you just write for the albuterol we will be all set." Larry was asleep in his mother's arms by this point in time.

It was not all snot and wheezes. It seems that for every two cute boogery kids, there was one that came in for their ADHD medication refill. In my opinion, this is an area of medicine that could be improved. Don't get me wrong. Dr. Wheeler and his partners seemed to be doing well in this regard, and were treating their patients appropriately based on the information they received. That is all you can ever do. But I always have to wonder with each ADHD kid whether they really do have the disorder, or if the problem lies with teachers and/or parents who don't have the time and energy to meet the child's needs without the crutch of pharmacology. Virtually all it takes for the diagnosis is a report from the teacher that little Billy can't focus in class, that he is disruptive, and mom and dad seeing the cycle continue at home when he can't focus there and the homework stacks up. At least some of this behavior is due to kids being kids, certainly toward the end of the day when they just want to do anything but be in a classroom. I hate to stand on a soapbox, but it seems to me I could have been labeled ADHD as well, but instead a nun smacked me with a ruler, told me to shut up, and pointed at my math problems. Problem solved. These patients were the most time consuming and difficult to deal with on this rotation.

When I was a student, a single group of drugs was used—all stimulants plus one non-stimulant. Now there is another "helper" drug you can add to the primary drug. When I was with Dr. Wheeler there was not yet a helper drug and the non-stimulant choice was not available in generic form. Every patient had to be seen before their controlled substance prescription could be refilled via a hand-carried written script. I was rather proud of Dr. Wheeler the few times he said no to starting one of these drugs, either because the child was acting calmly in the office and the story was not that bad (i.e., medicine wasn't necessary) or because the child was not yet in school and so was acting as any four- or five-year-old child would outside of a structured environment. This was no pill-mill, that was for certain. Fortunately for me, due to the difficulty and length of the visits and really needing to get it right the first time, I just tagged along and did not have to present any bouncing-off-the-wall patients to my preceptor.

One that stands out was eight-year-old third-grader, William, who came in because his dosage was not quite enough to get him to sit still at school, and it was quite apparent during the whole visit. The kid was like a BB in a balloon. I think his butt landed in his chair twice the whole visit, although he did spend a fair amount of time sitting in the middle of the floor making truck noises with a monster truck. "*Vrooooooooooooooom!*"

"So Mrs. Franklin, how have the mornings been?" Dr. Wheeler began the visit and did his best to shoot questions in between engine revs, and then listen to the answers that came during them.

"*Vroom!*"

"Well he takes his medicine, and usually it takes about an hour to kick in, so we know the start of the day will not be great, but we try to time it so it is in his system by the time he is dropped off."

"*Vroooooom!*"

"But even at that, it seems like he has some trouble, and by the end of the day it has all worn off. It's like it isn't even there."

"*Vroooom!*"

William was meeting with us about 4 p.m., so that explained the monster truck rally.

"Well he is on a pretty low dose, and only in the morning. We do like to taper up slowly, so we can go two directions."

"*Vroooooom!*"

"We can increase his morning dose or we can add a noontime dose to get him through the day. I would recommend we go higher, and then if he still needs a noontime nudge, we can give him the original low dose and go from there."

By this point in the visit, William was staring at a vaccination poster like it was a portal to another dimension, but only for a minute, before his mother brought him back and asked him to sit down for thirty seconds.

After the recommendation, Dr. Wheeler wrote a new script for a higher morning dose, and the nurse clipped a card to it to show the receptionist to schedule an appointment in one to two months. William went out the door and down the hall like bullet. His poor flustered mother, hair slightly mussed, calmly thanked us, strode steadily down the hall, and tried to locate her son. The visit almost made me feel twitchy inside.

The entire rotation was wonderful, thanks to a friendly preceptor as well as a fun patient population. I must include the hospital down the road, the one from my ortho rotation with—have I mentioned—the best doctor's lounge in all of town? I ate in style every day that rotation, without fail. With my choices for lunch being: drive to a fast-food restaurant, drop my own coin, and elevate my cholesterol; have a crappy sack lunch; or head over there for lunch in the lounge, it was an easy choice to make. I would have felt guilty, but it is not like Dr. Wheeler didn't have privileges there; it is the hospital where our RSV case was sent. Besides, the staff was used to seeing students and had already seen me. They always cook too much anyway. After the wonderful rotation with Dr. Wheeler and free hot lunches, it was time to head to the other side of town for my hematology-oncology rotation with one of the best lecturers from the didadic phase of our education. It was his kind mannerisms and soft-spoken personality, as well as my history working in a flow cytometry lab, that led me to request him as a preceptor on my second-to-last elective rotation.

Hematology/Oncology
Lincoln, Nebraska

I had just returned from a job interview at Mayo Clinic in Minnesota when I started my Hematology/Oncology rotation. Interestingly enough, it was in Rochester that I learned that things with a classy reputation do not always turn out to be a good personal fit when you get to experience them first hand. No matter, because I was not offered the position. The weekend was tumultuous, and not only because I had to fly in super early Saturday morning to start my rotation. Suffice it to say that due to a severe personal issue that arose Saturday night, the two weeks I spent with Dr. Harrison in Heme/Onc are somewhat of a blur. I will tell you, I wish my attention had not been on personal matters those two weeks; I would have gained so much more.

Dr. Harrison is one of the best preceptors in Lincoln, and despite my personal life reducing my time with him, he made the rotation rewarding and beneficial. He had suffered a stroke the year or so prior to me meeting him (don't quote me, I cannot recall the specifics) which left him with no real use of his right arm. During the two days he lectured us during the didactic phase, you could not tell. In fact, he arrived a bit late the first day and dived straight into his presentation. Throughout the lecture, he would take his right arm in his left and place it in his pocket or rest it on the podium, or he would walk about just as any other lecturer would. He moved his right arm with his left so seamlessly, as he had become accustomed to doing constantly, that no one noticed. It was only during our break at the top of the hour that he explained that he had suffered a stroke and that was why he wasn't using his right arm. I was impressed with how he had adapted so well that it was virtually undetectable. For this reason, plus my experience in Heme/Onc, I was one of the first to ask him (during the next break) if I could schedule an elective rotation with him. He gladly obliged.

I spent the first day of the rotation in Dr. Harrison's routine office on the east side of town. I parked and weaved my way through the waiting room and a few patient wings to the back where Dr. Harrison had a cluttered desk waiting for me. He apologized for the mess. "No one else here gets a scribe, but since I can't type anymore—at least, not at a productive speed—I have my own nurse who comes in with me on visits and types up the notes, or types them up from dictations on my tape recorder. That is her desk, but for a few weeks I told her she can share as long as you don't get in her way."

I understood completely and set my things down beside the desk. I really just needed the chair anyway. Dr. Harrison completed some dictations from the day before, and then his nurse, Stacey, arrived and it was time to begin seeing patients in clinic. Many providers see new patients in thirty-minute blocks and established patients in fifteen-minute blocks. Due to his condition, as well as the number of questions expected because of the patients' condition, Dr. Harrison saw new patients in hour blocks and established patients in thirty-minute blocks. This, in my opinion, only enhanced his bedside manner and clinical skills, since he was patient and took time to answer questions and properly care for the patients.

The first patient was established and about to start her second round of chemotherapy for breast cancer. Karen was in her early forties when a routine mammogram found a mass in her left breast. A needle biopsy by the primary care provider showed the mass to be malignant. Luckily for Karen, her tumor was HER2 (human epidermal growth factor receptor 2) positive, which meant there were additional, special drugs that target this cancer specifically and give the health care team another target to fire at when trying to kill the cancer. She had completed her first round of radiation and chemotherapy, which had shrunk the tumor prior to surgery with radiation and chemotherapy. Step two was to remove the tumor, and in her case, due to the number of lymph nodes the cancer had spread to, remove her entire breast via mastectomy. She was now ready for her second round of chemotherapy, followed by treatment with trastuzumab, the drug that would specifically target the HER2 receptor for any residual cells that had escaped the war against her cancer.

When we entered the room, Karen was already on the exam table with her husband in a chair across the room. Both were happy to see Dr. Harrison. Dr. Harrison introduced me, and then got right down to business. "So are you ready for round two?"

"I think so. I just can't wait to be done with all this, put it in the past. The chemo makes me so sick. It makes me want to get it over with and be a survivor, or die trying to survive because that is what the chemo does, makes you feel like you are dying while trying to survive."

Dr. Harrison grimaced and set the chart down. "I have to be honest with you, round two is usually worse, but it really does help by getting any stray cells that survived the first round and surgery. The good news is that the trastuzum-ab therapy is much better."

Tears welled up in Karen's eyes. "I want to get better, and I want to do whatever is necessary. Let's just do it and get it over with. The sooner the better."

Dr. Harrison went over the specifics of the second round of chemothera-py and proceeded to the physical exam, mostly cursory in nature, listening to Karen's heart and lungs, feeling around her stomach and listening there, and finally checking her ankles for swelling. Afterward, we marched down the hall, single file, to the outpatient IV treatment clinic where Karen would receive her next round of chemo.

"I know you know where to go Karen, but I wanted to show Sean here where the treatment takes place." Dr. Harrison showed me around. We peeked in on a few patients hooked up to bags, most of whom were either bald or wearing kerchiefs to hide their baldness, because hair loss is the most visible side effect of the drugs they were receiving. The drugs attack the dividing cells in the body; tumor cells divide quickly, but so do the cells that produce hair, and so these are a casualty of the treatment. Every patient had an emesis basin with them, since nausea and vomiting are also common during treatment. Luckily, each treatment room also featured a television, which took the patient's mind off the unpleasant task at hand.

The second half of my first day and all of my second day was spent at the East Lincoln clinic with Dr. Harrison. Here we saw mostly follow-ups similar to Karen, or patients on the hematology side of the specialty. Some had a can-cer of one blood cell line or another, either leukemia or lymphoma, but others had a hematological problem of another sort that was not cancerous.

An example of this was the young African American woman named Sandra whom we saw on day two. Sandra suffered from sickle cell anemia, a hematological disorder where under certain conditions her red blood cells take on a sickle shape, which makes it more difficult for them to carry oxygen. Even worse, with their jagged shape making them prone to getting caught in small arterioles, the disease can cause an impressive amount of pain. These ep-isodes can be caused by various stressors including weather changes, a woman's monthly cycle, and stress in general, though as is common with many disorders, the stressor is often not identifiable. This was poor Sandra's case, because her sickle cell exacerbations did not seem linked to anything in her life, but would just hit her out of the blue. This led her to need to utilize the ED over week-ends, late in the evenings, etc. Also, as I mentioned before, drug seekers are frowned upon and it is difficult to tell who is a seeker and who is legit. Anyone using the ED at a high frequency for pain is going to come under scrutiny. In fact, some EDs I have worked in will not allow the dispensing of narcotics out of the ED—only a single dose and a hand-carried script. For this reason, it was easier for Sandra to see Dr. Harrison for refills of her medication.

"Last week was pretty rough. About three days in a row I had to take my pain pills four times throughout the day. I am down to five, so I don't think I will make it through my next episode."

"I see, it looks like we filled your script just over a month ago. The pharmacy wants to see these scripts last a month or longer. I just mention that because I don't want them giving you a hard time."

Dr. Harrison leafed through Sandra's chart. "Make sure you are taking your hydroxyurea. It will help these episodes to occur further apart, maybe even for a shorter time."

"I will try. Trust me, I don't want to use the hydrocodone, but I don't want the pain. I take my daily meds religiously. Thanks, though."

Unfortunately, there is no cure for sickle cell disease. The closest we have come to a cure is to give the patient a transfusion of blood from another, sickle cell–free, individual. This dilutes the defective hemoglobin with healthy hemoglobin. The healthy blood cells live longer, and since they work better and for longer the body will make less defective hemoglobin for a bit. Due to the risks and complications, including that of iron overload, this intervention is reserved for the most critical of patients with the worst episodes, and usually only if the disease has led to an anemia. The body, specifically the spleen, often gets riddled with sickle cells, because its main job is to filter out diseased cells. If the spleen is very effective in filtering out diseased cells, the production of new cells may not keep up, which can lead to an anemic state. It can also be a source of severe pain if it becomes filled with these jagged cells. Thus, an extreme intervention in the disease is removal of the spleen. Dr. Harrison wrapped up the visit explaining this possibility if Sandra's disease continued to progress, and he sent her on her way with a new script for her next acute episode.

On Wednesdays and Fridays Dr. Harrison went to his West Lincoln clinic on the lower level of a specialty clinic closer to the new, and more affluent, part of town. In this clinic, the four days I spent with Dr. Harrison were taken up by oncology follow-ups and a few leukemias. One old farmer from this clinic springs to mind. Randal was sixty-four when he was diagnosed with Chronic Mylogenous Leukemia (CML). He had been able to push through the long days and hard work required in the combine at the end of summer corn harvest, but one year, out of the blue, he found himself feeling worn out by mid-afternoon. For a few days, he even had to leave the work to his sons and hired hands while he headed home to rest. He chalked it up initially to getting old, but when he became more and more worn out with even less arduous tasks, he went to see his primary care provider. A simple blood count showed that his white blood cell count was over twice what was expected (outside of an impressive infection) and was made up mostly of immature neutrophils (which are of the myeloid cell line, hence the M in CML). Randal was sent to Dr. Harrison's practice where a bone marrow biopsy confirmed the disease process suspected. Randal was started on imatinib, a drug from a class of pharmaceuticals that has virtually revolutionized the fight against the disease. Classified as a tyrosine kinase inhibitor, and thus a neoplasm inhibitor, this drug and the ones that followed almost doubled the survivability of CML. Thanks to catching the disease early, quick diagnosis, and intervention, Randal was back to full strength and farming as usual by the time the next harvest season rolled around.

As we entered the room he set his magazine down and shot to his feet. "Mornin' Doc. Who's your pal?" Randal shook both our hands as Dr. Harrison introduced Sean, his shadow. "A baby Doc, huh? Well good fer you. Keep up the hard work. I know it ain't easy, but if you've made it this far, you must be doin' something right!"

Dr. Harrison settled into his chair to review Randal's most recent blood count. "Randal wasn't this boisterous when I first met him. He looked like a bus had run him over."

"Felt like it, too!" Randal settled onto the exam table, but I could tell it was only because it was routine and not because he felt like settling down anywhere except maybe on his tractor seat.

"Your blood work looks excellent. Everything is normal. All your neutrophils are mature. No immature blast cells[6] at all."

"I feel as fit as a fiddle, all thanks to you, Doc."

"Well, I do what I can. Let me listen to you here." Dr. Harrison gave Randal his exam, certified him as, indeed, fit as a fiddle, and set him free to return to the farm to hit the ground planting or harvesting. Maybe both. Despite being raised in Nebraska, I am not familiar with farming in February.

I was fortunate during my time with Dr. Harrison to not experience any acute leukemias. There has not yet been any revolutionary drug to date that has increased survivability of the acute leukemias, and for this reason, when found in adults, the outcome is often grim. Randal was fortunate that he had developed a chronic leukemia. Had he developed Acute Mylogenous Leukemia (AML), the most common acute leukemia of adulthood, he likely would not have fared as well. Even when found in a younger person, survival is a flip of a coin at best. According to UpToDate, a website I use often to stay up to date, when caught in the teens, survivability of AML at five years is 53% and drops

---

6   The earliest identifiable stage of a blood cell. Typically, these stay in the bone marrow and mature, thus the presence of any in the blood stream is a sign that investigation is needed.

to 49% when found over age twenty-five. Survivability at age forty to fifty-nine is 33%; at age sixty to sixty-nine it is 13%; at age seventy to seventy-nine it is 3%; and over age eighty there are no survivors at five years.

Chronic leukemias are rare in children; the most common oncological disorder in kids is Acute Lymphocytic Leukemia (ALL), and luckily it has a survival rate at ten years of almost 90%, according to UpToDate. Despite this good outcome, I don't know if I could have handled pediatric oncology, coming right off my pediatrics rotation. I consider myself fortunate that the kids I saw during this rotation were mostly sickle cell or had some other fairly benign condition that would not dreadfully shorten their lives. In fact, the only exposure I have had to a young person with acute leukemia came a year prior to beginning PA school. I was privy to the case the morning after the evening shift at Creighton University Medical Center diagnosed a freshman on campus with ALL. This, of course, led to extra blood slides being made so that the patient's cells could be seen by other clinical laboratory scientists who wanted to sharpen their skills at the microscope. I came to learn that while I was looking at his cells, the young man in question was already at the oncologist scheduling his bone marrow biopsy to confirm the diagnosis, and finding out the treatment plan, including lymphocyte cell sites that could be targeted.

My final day with Dr. Harrison was, of course, bittersweet. I was looking forward to my next rotation, where I would perform two rotations back to back (or coinciding, as I saw it). I still had two to go, but only one more clinical site and only one more clinical team. I had greatly enjoyed my time, albeit brief, with Dr. Harrison. Luckily, there was a wonderful clinical team to be found as I returned to my old stomping grounds, and the scene of the lab story from above: Creighton University Medical Center.

Trauma/Emergency Medicine
Omaha, Nebraska

It felt odd to walk into the same hospital where I had been employed only a few years earlier. In fact, the lab is only a matter of feet from the hospital lobby and the elevator bay I would take up to the emergency department on the second floor. Naturally, I made sure I arrived at the hospital about thirty minutes prior to when I was expected in the emergency department so I could stop by the lab and say hello to my former co-workers. Hell hath no fury like a former labbie who hears you were in the building and did not say hello. After discussing my recent endeavors with people who were proud of me for chasing my dream of entering patient care, and dodging the icy stares of those who thought I had abandoned the lab for riches and fame, I proceeded up the stairs to the emergency department. CUMC is different from most hospitals in that its ED is not on the first floor. The first floor is typically chosen because it makes most sense; you can literally roll into the hospital if you are dying and be quickly carried into a treatment room. When they built CUMC, there was an idea of having a ramp off interstate 480 go right up into the parking lot of the ED, and it made sense to ramp over the local street traffic to expedite arrival. I still think it is a wonderful idea, but it never came to fruition. No matter, because there is a ramp off of the local streets (and ample employee parking underneath as well as the Creighton University Dental School).

Upon arriving on the second floor, I found my way to the front desk and was instantly greeted and swept back to the central pod of the ED to wait for my preceptor. Allison, the most recent hire to the department, had only been out of school two years, but in those two years she had acquired a large amount of knowledge and a vast skill set. Working in the ED allows you to see just about everything once and many things hundreds of times a year.

"Welcome to Creighton University Med. Center ED. Are you in for a treat!" Allison led me to the doctors' lounge between the break room (with fridges for doctors and staff) and the two trauma bays reserved for car wrecks and other unnatural disasters. "Feel free to keep your bag in here. There is a mini fridge here for soda and such, but you will want to put your food in the other room where the fridges are larger. Feel free to look up anything in your books, though your computer and phone will certainly be faster, and in the ED faster is better."

We left the doctors' lounge and ran into Dr. Williamson, another of my preceptors and now quite the famed speaker at regional CME conferences, including the Nebraska Academy CME conference every spring. "Hey man, welcome, good to have you here. If you have any questions, you just ask. Allison here is great, but I worked ED in Chicago and if she hasn't seen it, I have seen it at least twice." He gripped my hand and shook it vigorously.

I am not going to lie; I was glad to have saved this long rotation for the end of my rotations. Not only was this going to be insightful, but thanks to wonderful preceptors it would be delightful. Allison helped me find a place at what became known as "white coat row," where the students set up shop at laptops provided by CUMC to log into the electronic medical record. CUMC has so many students flow through the hospital— many of whom are their own—that they have streamlined the student log-in process and by the time you arrive they have everything ready to go. Here is your log in. There is your patient. Sure enough, after settling in, getting signed in, and being shown the patient board with patient age, sex, and chief complaint, I was told to pick one and get the ball rolling on "meet 'em, treat 'em, and street 'em. If you can't do that, TURF 'em," meaning get them taken care of so the next patient can be cared for, and if they are too sick to treat acutely, transfer them to the department that can help them (someone else's turf).

"I think I will take the abdominal pain in 3," I boldly stated to Allison, who almost died laughing.

"Oh no, I would never do *that* to you! Abdominal pain is the million-dollar work up, and that is a female to boot. You are looking at a detailed history, detailed exam including a pelvic exam (which is an invasive look into the vagina, in this case performed by some guy she doesn't know), labs, an X-ray at the least, a CT with contrast to follow, most likely, and God only knows what else. I will take that. You go see the snotty little kid in 1."

As I quickly learned, the more distant rooms were reserved for the non-emergent patients. There were sixteen rooms in all spread out across the emergency department:

1	2	Waiting Room/ Reception			12
3	4		11		13
5	6	16	15	14	
7					

Nurses' Station

Break Room/ Doctors' Lounge

White Coat Row

| 10 | 9 | 8 | Trauma Bays | Ambulance Bay/ Back Door |

So if you were in rooms 1, 2, 11, or 12, we had no fears of you dying in the next twenty-four hours. Rooms 3, 4, 8, 9, and 13: we didn't think you were gravely ill but still had to prove it to ourselves. Rooms 5, 6, 7, 8, 9, 14, 15, and 16: we did have very deep concerns and wanted to keep a real good eye on you. Of course this was just a guide. When the ED was full you could have a cold and still land in room 15 if everyone in the ED at that moment was not gravely ill. Room 10 was its own special room; it rarely held a sober person. Occasionally, when there were no drunks available there would be a cut finger or other minor injury in there, since it had a locked cabinet with almost every sort of suture material. However, for the most part, room 10 was a large closet with various supplies, and if you had to step over a patient to get to these, at least the patient would be passed out sleeping it off.

I proceeded to my first emergency room patient, a six-year-old male with a fever and cough in room 1. I reviewed the nurse's assessment in the EMR, grabbed my notebook, and entered the room. It was hard to tell who my patient was as I viewed the scene before me. I guessed that the smallest one jumping on the bed was too young, but the two young gentlemen sitting in the chairs with suckers in their mouths were both likely suspects.

"Hello, my name is Sean. I am a physician assistant student. Which of you is Michael?"

Nobody said a word, not even mom (?) who was leaning against the wall, staring intently at her phone.

I stepped closer to my two candidates. "Are you Michael?" The first one looked at me, shook his head, and then went back to watching *Scooby-Doo* on television.

The bed jumper helped me out, though by now I thought I had it. "Michael! Michael! Michael!" He pointed at the patient in the chair next to Not-Michael.

The caregiver (mom?) awoke from her cell phone daze and piped up, "Yeah, he gots a fever."

I reviewed the vitals. Temperature 98.7. "He looks good now. Did you give him any Tylenol or Advil?"

"Naw, I don't gots that."

I knew either of these drugs would return his temperature to normal, and that he was normal. This was a bit of a curveball for day one of the ED. What I knew: he liked *Scooby-Doo* and suckers. He is afebrile with no known cause of his normality. The kid jumping on the bed will be on Ritalin in a few years. I gave Michael a cursory exam: heart, lungs, ears, nose, and throat. He had a snotty nose and a lollipop-induced blue tongue, but appeared fine to me. "Alright, I think he is OK now. If his fever does return, you can give him either Tylenol or Advil—anything that has acetaminophen or ibuprofen from the kids' section of the pharmacy."

"I need a prescription for that."

I felt as though I had been asked a question I didn't know the answer to. "I'm sorry, what?"

"If you give me a prescription, Medicaid pays for it. I need a prescription for his medicine."

She didn't take her eyes off her phone, until I laid this on her: "Neither of those drugs are prescription strength, so you don't need a script, and I am guessing both are under five dollars—"

"I ain't got five dollars!"

Excellent. "Alrighty. Well, as I said, I am just the student. I am not the final word. Let me run this little guy's story by my preceptor." I put on the friendliest smile I could muster. Mom (?) glared at me as I exited the room. It was nice to have this cop out, but I knew it wouldn't last.

I found Allison and told her about our young man in no apparent distress with a runny nose and no fever. "Yep, happens every day. I have my medical card, see me or see my kid, give us our script so Medicaid pays for it. Have a nice day. Wait, wait, was the kid eating Cheetos?"

"Uhhhhh, no. But he was eating a sucker."

"Ah, a sucker. Usually it is Cheetos. I can't say why, but I tell you what: Those things are a miracle for abdominal pain." Allison took the chart from me and proceeded to room 1. "Hello, how is little Michael doing in here?"

Snotty Michael looked down from *Scooby*. "OK." Back to *Scooby*. Mom glared at me. Allison performed the same exam and pulled out her script pad. Was she throwing me under the bus? "Do you need a work note?"

"I ain't gots no job."

"OK." Script pad went back into her pocket, thank heavens. "Well, this looks like just a little virus, no ear infection or anything like that. Sean is right that his fever will respond nicely to Tylenol. If he hasn't had any for a while we can give him some here."

"Fine, but I really need a script to get more."

"As Sean already told you, you don't need a script for this medicine. I know it isn't cheap but it is over the counter, so I can't help you there."

"Whatever." Suddenly the phone was in her pocket and all three young men were marching out the door in a stumbling herd. "Assholes!"

I was a bit taken aback, but Allison just smiled the same smile I had proffered earlier. As they cleared the lobby door, Allison added, "Don't worry, you will be called worse. This is just your first day." Patient greeted, treated, and streeted. It was back to the desk to chart the encounter.

Allison showed me on her screen how to open up the patient's electronic chart, add the complaint, the exam with diagnosis, and the treatment plan. "Next one is yours, by the way. I am still working on that abdominal pain. You are welcome."

The next patient I selected from the board really was sick. Abigail had been suffering from a cold just like little Michael, but she had an impressive fever, a cough that brought up nasty phlegm, and shortness of breath. The ED board read, "Room 5: 73F SOA cough." Her chart read, "100.1F/87% O_2 on room air/Resp 30 HR 88."

I entered the room just as she finished coughing green mucus into a Kleenex. "Oh, I am so sorry, honey. That's just nasty. I feel like a bus ran me over. Ooooooh Lordy."

My sweet little old lady panted through the nasal cannula the nurse had placed under her nose to give supplemental oxygen. Unlike Michael, Abigail appeared to be in some distress. The finger pulse oximeter sat on the counter so I placed it on her finger as I listened to her heart and lungs. As I placed the stethoscope to her chest, her heartbeat was almost indiscernible from the horrible sounds rattling around inside her lungs. With each breath there was not only a wheeze but also the coarse sounds of fluid bubbling in both lungs. I did find her heart by focusing on the background, despite the noise around it. It sounded perfect. As I opened my eyes after focusing on her heart, I glanced at the pulse oximeter: two liters of oxygen via nasal cannula had raised her oxygen level to 90%—not really impressive.

I continued my exam, and it actually appeared as if her viral cold had almost resolved; her nose was slightly runny, but not terrible, her throat was not red, and her ears were fine. "Well, I think an X-ray of your lungs is going to be helpful today, and we should probably run some lab work as well just to see how the other parts of your insides are doing."

"Alright, honey, I will wait here. Thank you so much for helping me." She grabbed my hand in both of hers. Then she let go and broke into another coughing fit. I went to find Allison and figure out how to order lab and X-ray.

Shortly thereafter, Abigail's chemistry and blood count lab results appeared in the computer. She had an elevated white blood cell count indicating infection, her electrolytes were all a bit off but nothing terrible; however, it was rather obvious from her results that she was having a difficult time exchanging air in her lungs.

Allison turned in her chair away from the computer. "I bet her chest X-ray looks like hell. Have you ever seen a white out?"

"Only in textbooks."

"Well, I have a feeling we are going to keep this one, so I will wait until that chest X-ray comes back. You have done all the work, while I get all the credit." Allison playfully punched me in the arm. As good as it felt to be helpful, my heart broke to know my little old lady in room 5 was as sick as she was. Moments later her chest X-ray came back. Sure enough, both lungs were virtually whited out by fluid accumulating in all five lobes: pneumonia. In a way I was kind of happy, because if the X-ray had come back showing just bronchitis, if her white count had not been so high, if her oxygen level had improved slightly after a coughing fit, we would have sent her home, but now we could admit her to the medical floor for care.

I followed Allison to room 5. "Good morning Abigail. Sounds like you are having a rough day."

"Oh Lord Jesus, I been feeling like hell for almost a week now, but today I just can't take it anymore." Tears welled up in her eyes.

"Well I have bad news and good news. The bad news is your labs confirm that you are one sick lady, and your X-ray is rather impressive. You have a nasty pneumonia going on, both lungs. How you just walked into my ED today is beyond me." Allison took Abigail's hands in hers. "But the good news is that we are going to find you a bed upstairs, get you some medicine, and get you feeling better. Do you have any family to call? Do you want anything brought from home?"

"Oh no, sweetie, it's just me. Leroy died years ago, and the children all live so far away. I have my cell phone. We can call them later, but they couldn't get here if they tried."

Allison patted Abigail's hands. "You just wait here. The nurses will be back with a wheelchair to take you upstairs shortly." Allison and I exited the room and I documented the visit, and then Allison showed me how to enter admission orders. "You students are great at SOAP notes. How are you at admission H and Ps?"

"I am pretty good."

"Excellent! Have at it, slugger!" Allison clicked a few times and the H and P template appeared on the screen. "I will call medical and get her a bed reserved."

The rest of my first day was uneventful, but I knew that the next day would likely not be so quiet (a word that, by the way, is banned from use in the ED because the instant someone utters the Q-word all hell breaks loose). Creighton and UNMC, the University of Nebraska Medical Center, take turns on trauma coverage. The ownership of hospitals in Omaha has changed so much since I lived there that this may no longer be the case, but when I worked there, and as a student, CUMC took trauma coverage on Tuesday, Thursday, and Saturday and UNMC took it the other days. Day two, Tuesday, was certain to be full of excitement.

On my first week I had drawn the 7 a.m. to 7 p.m. coverage, and luckily enough for me, trauma coverage begins at 7 a.m. As is likely typical in any metropolitan area, it does not take long before someone gets in trouble on their morning commute, complicating the day for of hundreds of people, but worst of all, injuring themselves and/or others in a motor vehicle accident (MVA). By the time I had completed my commute from my friend Stephen's house, where I was staying, a thirty-six-year-old female had not checked her blind spot on the interstate and had clipped another car driven by a forty-seven-year-old female. The EMTs radioed ahead the details and vitals of our two patients, just as I settled in at my computer to sign in. Due to the non-secure nature of the transmission, we are not given names, and so off the printer came paperwork and ID bands for Jane Doe 1 and Jane Doe 2. So, due to the frantic pace of the ED/trauma bays, these two ladies were known as: one and two.

As we waited in the trauma bay, Allison told me we would take whichever one arrived second. Neither patient sounded all that terrible, but this way I could see how things went before I had to participate. Thus, two teams formed, one in each trauma bay, consisting of a doctor, PA, phlebotomist, X-ray tech, two nurses, and an EMT.

One and two both arrived at almost the same time so Allison and I just stepped over to trauma bay two and listened to the presentation from the EMT on the ambulance crew. "This is our thirty-six-year-old female driving the front car in a lane-change collision, her left rear vs. car two right front panel, car spun

180 before striking median facing wrong direction. Fully restrained, air bags deployed, remained in position throughout. Mild facial lacs likely secondary to airbag, complaints of left shoulder pain at scene, denies neck pain/abdominal pain/back pain. Alert and ambulating at the scene, agrees to transport for assessment and treatment as necessary, she is all yours."

Dr. Williamson was taking the report on the other victim. Allison and I stood next to his partner, Dr. Atul, who nodded in agreement. "Very good, thank you gentleman very much. Young lady how are you feeling? Is that still a good assessment of your complaints? Is there anything new?"

"Well . . . to . . . tell you the truth . . . now that I have been lying on this board . . . my back hurts, but I really do think it is just this stupid board. Are you guys going to get rid of it soon?"

"Let me check you over first, young lady." Dr. Atul began his head-to-toe assessment, checking her neck, back, abdomen for pain, heart and lungs, eyes, ears, nose, and throat, and he moved her legs about. "Yes, you appear to be in decent enough shape. Nurses let us move her off the backboard."

"Sean, today you are a nurse. Get in there." Allison gave me a nudge, and there I was, at the bedside, in the trauma bay, helping with a MVA.

Luckily, actual nurses are super helpful and one of them gave me the easy job in the process. "I tell you what, come over here, and when we get her propped up you just pull the board." Sounded good enough to me.

As we laid her down, Dr. Atul rattled off his orders. "OK, let's get cranial films including ocular orbits, throw in a C-spine just to cover our asses, A/P and lateral of the left shoulder. Bring her back and we will go from there." Off he went to the doctors' lounge to await the films he had just ordered.

Allison stepped up beside me. "You want to stay here and clean her up, or move over and see how the other one is doing?" I was, of course, all about seeing as much as possible, so I suggested we see how the other patient was doing. She, unfortunately, had done far worse in the accident. Her car had flipped halfway over and she had hit her head on the driver's side door in the process. Not only was she strapped to the backboard, but she was in a cervical spine collar immobilizer, and she had a rather impressive laceration above her left eye to which a nurse was applying pressure while trying not to move the patient's head.

Right about the time I arrived an X-ray tech showed up to take the patient for a set of c-spine films that would show if all that cervical spine protection was necessary or not. By the time she was wheeled back, Dr. Williamson was reviewing the films of her head and neck and could verify that she had not fractured anything when she hit her head and could be moved into a more comfortable situation. The rollover patient had superseded the other patient, who was now in X-ray, so I was allowed to sew the head laceration of the rollover victim. I had treated at least a dozen lacerations by this point, but never had I done so with such a large audience. Dr. Williamson wanted a blood alcohol level on both patients and a CBC on the one I was sewing, just in case her head wound had released a little too much blood. So, as I did my best to close up a head wound, the phlebotomist performed a blood draw, the X-ray tech hovered in the background to see if she was needed again, the nurses cleaned the more superficial wounds, and Allison watched to make sure I was doing alright.

Then the patient's family arrived. They were not allowed to hang out in the trauma bay and were quickly escorted to the waiting room. Still, this was the first time I was in the middle of sewing when an emotional husband came in crying as I helped fix his wife. The best part of the story is that the X-rays on the thirty-six-year-old came back clear, and once all the abrasions and cuts were cleaned both patients were declared to be in no grave danger. And before lunch they were both released with only cuts and bruises.

Later that afternoon I picked a very interesting patient off the board. The description read, "50M abdominal distension and pain." I hadn't been around very long, but I figured I could not hide from the million-dollar work up forever; it was time to tackle an abdomen. Plus, it was a male patient so no need for a pelvic exam. Allison agreed that I could try and she would help me through it. Besides, after helping on a double trauma on only my second day, it would be nice to settle into a quiet investigation. There was still the possibility that another nasty trauma would come in and pull both Allison and I away, and this was a case that would allow me to step away and assist in the trauma without any great detriment to the patient.

I will never forget the smell or the scene before me as I entered that exam room. I was almost knocked over by the smell of alcohol and marijuana that came wafting at me as I opened the door. Most impressive about this stench was that inside the exam room nobody was smoking or drinking. There was just a little yellow man with bloodshot eyes and the abdomen of a starving African child. His name was Leroy. "Before you say anything, there is no way you are going to get me to stop drinking or toking." The little yellow man with the big belly welcomed me before I could introduce myself. "I've heard it all before and there isn't anything more you can say to get me to change my mind."

"Alrighty then. Well, I am Sean, a PA student here. Let's start with your alcohol and marijuana use. How much do you think you use of each on any given day?"

The little yellow man had calmed down. "I drink about a case, and probably only three or four bowls per day. The marijuana, usually in the morning, helps clear my head from the day before, you know."

I did not know, but I jotted this down anyway. "And how many years do you think you have been using each?"

"Oh, I've been using weed for over thirty years, been drinking a little longer than that, but I only got up to a case a day these last fifteen or so."

My thought was that he had likely consumed a brewery's daily production, but I kept that to myself. I continued asking him questions about his health and history. He had been diagnosed with severe cirrhosis a few years back, but even this had not stemmed his alcohol use. He was quite aware that it was killing him, and he said he prayed for death every day as he poured beer down his throat, but despite this there was no way he could quit, even if he tried. In fact, by this point, he figured the damage was done and what good would quitting be anyway?

"Truthfully doc, all I want today is for you guys to get this fluid off my gut, get me something for the itching and the pain, and let me go home to die."

I knew better than to try to do anything more than "treat 'em and street 'em" but figured we should at least run some labs to see how bad off he was. I finished the initial visit with his physical exam, including thumping his distended abdomen, which sounded like a ripe watermelon ready for harvest. I found Allison and ran my treatment plan by her: IM[7] Benadryl for the itching, chemistries to assess his disease state, PT/PTT to see if his liver was making any clotting factors whatsoever, and though I could not do it, if it would make the patient feel better, find someone in house who could perform a paracentesis to remove the fluid from his abdomen. This was indeed possible, but we would have to admit the patient to the medical floor for this procedure. I informed Allison that I doubted we would succeed in getting this guy to stick around; she agreed it would be difficult. We both agreed to wait until the labs confirmed how sick he was before trying to state our case, because we expected that the labs would reinforce our argument. Not surprisingly, his liver enzymes were through the roof, as was the amount of time it took for his blood to clot on the coagulation testing when his lab results came back. Furthermore, he was malnourished and lacking in all of his electrolytes.

I ordered a banana bag to be hung (an IV infusion containing thiamine, folic acid, and magnesium), and after it had infused for about an hour I approached the patient about the possibility of paracentesis if he would stay in the hospital at least overnight. "Have the Benadryl and fluids helped with the itching?"

"Little bit, yeah. I feel better."

---

7   Intra-muscular, injected into a muscle, usually the thigh.

"Excellent, but we can make you feel even better if you will let us. We can have a surgeon remove the fluid from your abdomen. We want to make sure we get the needle in the right spot. This is especially important because I checked your ability to form a clot in response to injury, and it was not very impressive. If the needle nicks anything during the process we need to be able to fix that quickly as well. Of note, your liver enzymes were through the roof, but I doubt this is of any surprise to you."

"Not really. I mean, I'm yellow. My liver is more than shot."

"True, very true. The thing is, to do that procedure we will have to keep you overnight. The surgeons are all busy with scheduled cases. They can do it later this evening, but we need to watch you afterward for a few hours, so overnight would be best."

Leroy adamantly disagreed with this treatment plan and demanded that the procedure be done and he be discharged or not be done at all. I did not want to admit defeat just yet, so I agreed to see if it could be done sooner on an outpatient basis. Allison sighed deeply, rubbed her eyes, and agreed to try. She was able to get a surgeon who was not too busy to agree to do a modified paracentesis, where he would remove some of the fluid but would not put the needle into Leroy's abdomen deep enough to get all of it. To quote him: "Doesn't matter how much we take off, it's coming right back anyway." This statement was quite true. We added some lactated ringers to the IV set and transferred Leroy's care to the surgeon. He would be back to swilling and toking that very afternoon, just as he wanted.

Some days it seemed as if there were trends or "runs" in the emergency department. Shortly after wrapping up Leroy's case, the scanner went off notifying us that an ambulance was inbound with a thirty-year-old male in police custody after causing a scene in one of the seedier areas of town. Then the paramedics added that he was on PCP and that he was still giving them a difficult time.

Allison got way too excited. "Oh, it's your lucky day! Have you ever seen anyone on PCP? It's crazy!"

"I can honestly say that I have not."

"Well, we will see if he has calmed down. If so, you can take a good look at him. I will go get the benzos ready to calm his ass down."

I could hardly contain my delight; I just hoped they had strapped this tweaker down really tight. Luckily, by the time he rolled in on his gurney he was still seeing a whole other world but was calmer about it and was indeed strapped down tight. I cannot remember what he was saying as he rolled in and cannot concoct anything even close to what he was experiencing. All I do recall, is that in his world I was an alright guy and was allowed to examine him. His heart was racing, his breathing was rapid (despite his lungs being clear), and his pupils were blown. That was the most impressive part of the whole exam. I shined my pocket light into both of his eyes and his pupils did not constrict one bit. I'd had my pupils dilated by my eye doctor before and could not take him shining the light into my eyes for even a second, but this gentleman stared at my light as if it were something he had never seen before, perhaps a whole new world opening up before his dilated eyes. I couldn't believe it. I joked to Allison that this would be a perfect time for an eye exam (and, truth be known, I did come back with the ophthalmoscope to look at the back of his eye, because when an opportunity like this presents itself you don't let it slip by). She agreed, but doubted he would follow-up to pick up his lenses.

My first week was fairly unremarkable as it wound down: a few runny noses, a laceration or two, a few drunks sleeping it off. On my second week I had to cover 7 p.m. to 7 a.m. I was A: scared of what happens in the ED overnight and B: less than thrilled as I am definitely not a night-time kind of guy and knew my body would never really get used to these hours, and if it did I would adapt just in time to go back to daytime shifts.

I showed up my first night after having tried to sleep that afternoon without success. I brought what Taco Bell would call a fourth meal so that I didn't starve to death in the middle of the night, and settled in for my adventure. The evening got off to a nice enough start—same old problems—and then Bernice rolled in. I had no idea who she was, but everyone else seemed to be old pals with her. She came in via ambulance as someone had found her passed out on a curb downtown and called 9-1-1. She was alert and chatty when she arrived and was escorted straight to room 10 to sleep it off. I didn't think about her much; she was just another drunk. I had a patient to document after having diagnosed her strep throat, written a script for penicillin, and discharged her.

I was documenting the physical exam when I sensed a presence to my right. It was Bernice. "Well, aren't you a sexy little doctor? Who's your friend?" I followed her gaze to the M1 student, Mark, on my left.

We both sat there uncomfortably for a few seconds until Dr. Atul, the overnight physician, noticed and chased her off. "Leave those poor students alone! Back to your room Bernice!"

"Hey, the heart wants what it wants." She winked and stumbled back to her room for ten minutes. Then she was back. "So I see you are married. Do you swing?"

"Bernice! Room!" Dr. Atul rose out of his chair, and I half expected him to grab a broom and shoo her like a cat off a porch. The third time she came out, Dr. Atul had had enough. "That's it. If you can flirt with the students you are sober enough to leave. I'm calling the police to pick you up." Shortly thereafter, the police arrived and escorted their public intoxication "suspect" off in little silver bracelets.

Eventually, things calmed down. Since we were not on trauma call, the few things that did trickle in were fairly benign. Dr. Atul thought it wonderful that he had two students to cover the ED and took the opportunity to sleep in the doctors' lounge in a recliner. He slept soundly as Mark and I managed the few things that did come in, but at about 6 a.m. the flow increased and we had to wake him up for more than just signing off on a treatment plan. I was the one to wake him for the day in order to tell him about our abdominal pain: Becky.

Of course, no one wanted an abdomen when they were only an hour away from going home, but someone had to take it, so I jumped in. I introduced myself to the poor woman curled up on the bed and proceeded to document her story. The pain had begun in the middle of the night. She thought it was just indigestion. She stated that it was crampy all over and just about unbearable. She could not remember any bad food, her monthly cycle had ended two weeks prior, and no one else around her was sick. Her pain seemed to have come out of nowhere.

I examined her and no matter where I touched her abdomen she winced in terrible pain. Under the stethoscope, I heard nothing out of sorts. The rest of her exam was fine as well, though I couldn't comment on the pelvic since I had left that for Allison. In fact, all I did was order the CT with oral contrast and labs and then turf her off on Allison before heading home to attempt some daytime sleep. It wasn't until that evening, when I was coming back on, that Allison let me know that the labs were normal, the CT was normal, and that the patient had been given a GI cocktail (an antacid, lidocaine, phenobarbital, hyoscyamine, atropine, and scopolamine) and had been sent home with no real diagnosis. However, this would not be the last time I saw Becky; she appeared a total of four times during my six weeks at Creighton. Each time it was the same thing: normal labs, nothing telling on any imaging performed—CT or X-ray—and nothing telling on physical exam. Eventually, surgery was consulted to take out her appendix during an exploratory laparoscopy. The pathology report showed that the appendix was mildly inflamed; the surgical report itself stated that nothing was found while exploring her abdomen. Of course, this took place at the end of my rotation, so I do not really know what happened to her. She could still be going weekly to the CUMC ED, suffering to this day, and I just don't know it.

Sometime later that week—I have no shame admitting that the whole week was a sleep-deprived blur—we got good and deep into the bar scene. The first patient came in with a laceration on the ulnar or pinkie side of her left hand. Injuries to the ulnar side of the arm are sometimes known as "defensive wounds," often caused by the victim of an attack placing the arm in front of the face or above the head to deflect a blow. Boy, did this patient have a story.

When I entered the exam room she was in the middle of the story, which saved me a few questions during my eventual interview. "That bitch came at me screaming that I was trying to steal her man. I told her to step down and she tried to club me with her beer bottle. She's lucky I stopped her, but now I'm at the ER. Gonna get stitches."

I jotted down a few notes as she wrapped up her story and informed the other party she would have to call them back.

"So is that beer bottle the cause of your bloody hand this eve—" I glanced at my watch. "—morning?"

"Yeah, that bitch cray. She tried to kill me. I told the police she tried to kill me with that beer bottle. Probably woulda if I hadn't blocked it then popped her in the mouth!"

I didn't recall seeing any mouth poppings on the ED board so either the assailant didn't care, didn't feel it, or wound up at UNMC. Nonetheless, the laceration was rather impressive and was dripping on my exam room floor so I informed her we should cover it, get X-rays, and if there were no fractures I would gladly close it myself. She agreed this sounded acceptable, and I excused myself to order the films and wait. Luckily, about half an hour later her X-ray confirmed there was not any sort of problem other than the disruption of the skin on her hand and wrist. I gathered my local anesthesia and suturing supplies and re-entered the room to find her on the phone telling her impressive tale again. Eventually I got her to hang up and sit down so I could clean her hand. After doing so, and prepping the area with iodine and isopropyl alcohol, I placed a sterile paper drape around the affected area. Just then a nurse knocked on the door to let me know the patient's sister/ride home had arrived. I allowed her in. "Oh, my God, Janine. You should have saw it. That crazy bitch tried to kill me!" My patient jumped out of her chair, flinging my sterile drape through the air.

I put on my perturbed face and asked if she could please have a seat so I could sew her laceration.

"Oh, my bad."

After donning a new set of sterile gloves, and placing a new sterile drape, we began again. The entire time I was doing this the patient was telling her story to her new audience. I figured if this kept her seated and distracted it was a good thing. Two sutures later I learned otherwise; she was a hand talker. She leapt up to demonstrate how she had defended herself, raising the affected hand into the air, my suture and needle trailing like a kite tail. I walked over to the door and pulled it open with my elbow. "Nurse, can you help me in here?"

The nurse came in, and after we explained to the patient that she needed to remain still, the nurse took a hold of the patient's elbow to help her remember.

"My bad, my bad."

Her bad indeed. Eventually, I did manage to finish, thanks to my nurse who at least three times pinned the elbow to the procedure table, and the patient was discharged to regale the rest of Omaha with her tale.

Later that week I saw another bar-related injury, but this one was a much less intense battle: drunk guy versus tall curb. A forty-five-year-old convention attendee, a businessman from Canada, had just finished paying his bar tab when he walked out of the bar, misjudged the distance from the curb to the street, and landed flat on his face. Luckily, his glasses caught him; unfortunately, they penetrated the skin under his eyebrow, leaving blood streaming down his face. After I had introduced myself and gathered that information, I began the exam. He had managed to miss his nose, the bone under the laceration felt stable, and he checked out neurologically (except for the intoxication, of course), so I told him I could probably just sew him up and have him on his way in no time.

After gathering the necessary materials, I began to clean him up, and that was when he turned into quite a chatty gentleman. As I cleaned him up he told me his wife was probably going to kill him because he had used his white dress shirt to stop the bleeding. I saw it in the corner of the room and realized he was only wearing his sweater. Both looked like props from a slasher film.

"If I just leave it here, you could dispose of it. I doubt she will notice one dress shirt missing. I am lucky you guys are not too far from my hotel. I didn't even have to walk far after my little stumble. Say how much is this going to cost?"

"Actually, I don't know. I am not real well versed on the billing side of things. I just fix them up and send them home."

"Right, right, well I will inquire with your secretary up front and pay her on the way out."

I was a bit taken aback, "I am pretty certain if you gave her your insurance card, they will just send you a bill if you owe anything."

"Really? In Canada, it is at least twenty-five dollars for sutures like this."

I thought to myself, buddy you spent well over $25 just by walking in the door.

"I wouldn't worry about it, and I guarantee you if you leave a copy of your insurance card, whoever gets paid will make sure they find you."

"Alright then, that is just so different from what we have up north. Say, do you like hockey? I love the Red Wings myself, as far as the States goes, but for the most part I am a Maple Leafs fan."

As I closed his head wound I had to admit I was not much of a hockey fan. "I think there is a minor league team in the middle of Nebraska, the tri-cities something or another, but I am not much of a hockey fan. I enjoy football more. Football is real big here."

"Ah yes, you huskers of corn are quite fanatical, aren't you?" He started to chuckle, very much enjoying his own turn of phrase. "Did you know they have hockey in Arizona? That is just crazy, hockey in the middle of a desert."

Eventually, after discussing why it is weird that Americans call football soccer and what we play in the Super Bowl football, the sutures had been placed and he was on his way. Whether or not he gave the receptionist $25, I do not know.

During my week of overnights I stayed at my friend Stephen's house in Omaha, because I was afraid of falling asleep on the interstate to Lincoln and winding right back in the ED at Creighton on the wrong side of the stethoscope. I know I was at Stephen's house, I think I ate frozen dinners mostly, but to be honest I was just a zombie that came and went. My week of overnights was a haze of trying to stay awake all night, and then praying to fall asleep while the sun poured into his spare bedroom/office. In fact, the last thing I did before leaving for good was to bring Stephen and his wife, Adriane, small parting gifts, but Adriane's did not make it as sleepy Sean dropped the bottle of wine getting out of the car in their garage. It smelled like Bernice had stopped by.

That reminds me of the next time Bernice stopped by. I had been back on days for only a few days. Due to her history of harassing the male students, she was no longer allowed to remain in room 10. Besides, this time she had been brought in only because the ambulance drivers saw her walking down the middle of the street in front of the hospital and escorted her in. She was sober enough to go to the police department, but the EMT crew did not have time to drive her there. So Bernice was sent to room 1 with hopes she would behave herself there. She did not. Over the next ten to fifteen minutes I kept seeing her sneaking down the hall, the ward clerk chasing her back and closing the door, only for it to open a few seconds later. Eventually, two Omaha police officers strolled in. Looking back it was kind of like a movie starring Denzel Washington and Omar Epps. Bernice would have been played by Phyllis Diller. Nonetheless, I about fell off my stool laughing when fifteen seconds after the two officers cleared my view I heard Bernice exclaim, "Sweet Jesus, you sent me two sexy ones this time!" A minute later, there was Bernice between the two of them, grinning ear to ear, her fawning gaze bouncing between them trying to decide which one to pounce on first. I was just glad she had moved on from me, and no, it did not break my heart.

Later that week I met a patient with a broken heart, who just about broke my heart. Loretta had been in an abusive relationship for years and had become a regular in the ED at CUMC due to the abuse she endured at the hands of her live-in boyfriend. She came in via ambulance and looked like she had been in some sort of terrible accident or a war somewhere. Her white shirt was more blood red than white, her two front top teeth were held in her right hand, and she was crying profusely. Between sobs she exclaimed, "You call the police! That bastard is going to jail!"

The closest EMT sighed while his partner shook his head. "Loretta, are you really going to press charges? Because every time we call the police down here you change your mind, and then what . . . a few weeks go by, and here we are again."

"I'm gonna do it. You bring me the police!"

The lead EMT radioed back to dispatch to send a patrol over to CUMC for an assault inquiry, but he did not seem to believe it would be successful. "She is all yours. Same as usual, but this time he threw a brick at her."

With that, they were gone, and the nurse cleaned up our bloody victim. Like any nurse worth her salt, she was working not only on the exterior wounds, but some of the interior ones. "You know, Loretta, you don't deserve this. You deserve better. All you have to do is tell the police your story, tell them you want to press charges, and they will take care of it."

"Oh, I know, and today is the day!"

"Loretta, you say that every time. You really need to listen to me. He doesn't love you. This is not love. You need to be strong when the police arrive and remember that."

"Oh, I know, I know."

"Loretta, say it. Repeat after me: this isn't love."

"This ain't love. Oh, I know."

During their discussion I had recalled that if one were to get to a dentist quickly, often it was possible to re-implant teeth. The whole 'put it in a cup of milk and drive fast' idea. I figured I could do the same with Loretta's teeth. I informed the nurse of this as she finished cleaning up Loretta. She shook her head and laughed. "Good luck with that." The bleeding had stopped in Loretta's mouth and so, using gauze to get a good grip, I gently but firmly tried to implant the first tooth. It stayed. Success! I did the same with the second, and then the first tooth fell out. The nurse started to chuckle. "Son, even if you get those teeth to stay put, as soon as she leaves they are as good as gone."

I agreed, placed the teeth on the mayo stand[8], and went back to the physical exam. Other than her mouth, she was actually doing well. Her nose was not visibly broken or bleeding, ears nose and throat were healthy, and the brick apparently caught her straight on the mouth. I ordered X-ray to make sure nothing was broken and went back to my station to document everything.

Shortly after she returned from X-ray, and while I was reviewing her films (all normal), the police cruiser pulled up. The officers strolled in, inquired as to the whereabouts of the assault victim, and proceeded to her room.

Moments later a commotion broke out. "Oh, lord, no. I can't press charges! He can change. I know he can!"

A few nurses shook their heads as Allison and I proceeded to the exam room. Loretta was crying as one of the police officers patted her on the back and shook his head. "Loretta, we can't help you if you don't want help. I don't think anyone who throws bricks at other people during a discussion has any potential to change. We have been over this before, but there is nothing we can do if you don't give us the power to do something. We are handcuffed until you let us handcuff him."

Loretta started crying even harder. "I can't . . . I just . . ." Her words trailed off into her tears.

The police officer scribbled a few notes on his pad and put it away. "Last chance, Loretta. Do you want us to go arrest the son of a bitch?"

Loretta shook her head.

"Well, if you change your mind, here is my card. Call me, call 9-1-1, call a women's shelter, call anyone who can get you out of that house. I don't even care if you press charges as long as you get the hell away from that guy." The police officers nodded to me on their way out the door and were gone. Loretta placed the calling card on the mayo stand next to her teeth.

Later, after she was discharged, the nurse came out with the teeth and the card. "Want me to save these for her to pick up next week? Or just throw them out?" We threw them out. Neither the teeth nor the card were going to stick, and I didn't know which I found sadder. It took time to get over Loretta that day, but since I had many other patients to treat I had to, and so I found a way to move on.

Early the next morning, I had a patient who helped improve my mood after the previous day's gloom. It didn't seem as if she would cause any sort of mirth when I picked her off the board. In fact, I thought my whole day was shot. I think I might have picked her because I knew abdominal pain in a

---

8   A sideways U-shaped mobile stand designed for use in surgery where it can be placed over the patient maximizing space. They are used in the ED for laceration repair mostly, but since they are in every room they get used as a catch all.

forty-year-old woman would be the "million-dollar workup" and take all day, which would keep me busy and my mind off Loretta, who would one day likely die at the hands of her abusive lover. I walked into room 6 and shook the hand of a very prim and proper woman named Nancy who was sitting on the exam table. She appeared to be in no great pain but was not dressed as one would expect a drug seeker to be, so initially I was confused. I admit that I feel bad for stereotyping drug seekers, but at least at CUMC it was not the housewives that sought narcotics; it was usually a member of a lower rung on society's ladder. Nonetheless, I knew I would have to get a very detailed history and, seeker or not, the story would come out in due time.

"Hello, my name is Sean. I am a PA student. You are having abdominal pain. Can you tell me more about it, and how you would describe it, where it is located, how it started?"

"Actually, the problem is a bit lower." She unfolded her hands in her lap. "Do you know what Ben Wa balls are?"

Instantly, the song of the same name by Blink-182 started playing in my head. It was all I could do to not laugh, but amazingly I managed to hold off even a smirk and maintain professionalism. "Actually, I have and—"

"Kegel exercises. I was doing my Kegel exercises today. When I was done, I was unable to retrieve them."

"I see."

Luckily, she had interrupted me before I said something to embarrass both of us, because I had never heard of Ben Wa balls being used for anything besides a pleasurable experience.

"How long have they been in there exactly?"

"I would say an hour." She glanced at the gold watch on her wrist and then refolded her hands in her lap.

"This should be an easy fix, but as you can expect we will need you to disrobe from the waist down. I will grab the stirrup attachment for the bed, and due to the nature of the exam, my female preceptor, Allison, will assist me in getting things set up. I will give you enough time, and we will knock before coming in." I fetched a drape from a drawer under the bed and drew the curtain as I exited the room.

Allison looked up. "That was fast. You run into a problem?"

"Have you ever heard of Ben Wa balls?" Allison covered her mouth and did not succeed in stifling her laugh. I was glad I was the one who interviewed the patient.

"Oh, my god, no!"

"Yep, she put them in and cannot get them out." A few nurses wandered over, and some of them had no idea what we were talking about. Allison opened her web browser and did a quick search because they could hardly believe that such a thing existed. As the images popped up, the nurses started chuckling to themselves or stood with their mouths agape. It was soon apparent that some models of Ben Wa balls come with a retrieval string that holds the pair together; our patient's did not. Allison, a nurse, the bed extension, and I re-entered the room (after knocking) and I introduced my colleagues to the patient. After we got the bed pieced together, Nancy slid her feet into the stirrups and scooched into the proper position for the pelvic examination. Gently and professionally I eased her into the exam and placed the speculum in her vagina. I advanced the speculum until her cervix came into place. Everything appeared normal, which was good, but I was worried about the location of the foreign objects. "Move a little to the left," Allison whispered in my ear. I moved the end of the speculum to the left (the patient's right) and *floomp*, one Ben Wa ball slid into the speculum and rolled side to side. I tiled the speculum handle down, the first ball fell out, and I handed it to the nurse. On a hunch, I pulled the speculum back a bit, around the cervix and to my right (patient's left), and *floomp*, Ben Wa ball two slid into the speculum and rolled side to side. A tilt of the handle and out came ball two, which I handed to the nurse. Before withdrawing the speculum, I asked, "There are only two, right? 'Cause I found two."

"That is correct." As she confirmed this, up popped her right hand with a small silk bag.

"This is their carrying case. After you clean them, please return them to their satchel."

I cleaned her up a bit, removed my gloves, and took the bag from her to give to the nurse who was at the sink, her shoulders shaking gently. As I approached her, I realized she was doing her best not to laugh. It was funny, but only because the patient was not sick, was not injured, was just in an embarrassing situation. I think what made it even funnier though, was that she was not at all embarrassed. She was composed the whole time, as if getting Ben Wa balls stuck in one's vagina was to be expected from time to time.

The following day was my second-to-last day at Creighton and my last trauma day. I had seen a few car wrecks, I had helped a guy who had fallen off a ladder and shattered his pelvis, but while in house I had been a talisman that warded off traumas. That ended sometime on my last trauma day. Late in the afternoon, I witnessed one of the most gruesome injuries I had seen in person, even to date. It is likely that many viewers of YouTube or Rob Dyrdek's *Ridiculousness* have seen such injuries occur, but never the aftermath. A sixteen-year-old male high school student was brought in after missing the landing on his BMX bike during what was described by his friends later on as a "bad-ass jump." When he came down, virtually all of his weight was thrown onto his right leg as it hit the edge of the steps he was flying over. After he spilled onto the ground, his buddies took one look at his right ankle and called 9-1-1 immediately. His right foot was broken and flipped to the outside, and he needed medical help.

The paramedics brought him in, and he was quickly escorted to trauma bay 1. I arrived with Allison to watch, and Dr. Williamson took over. Before the double doors could swing closed behind him, Dr. Williamson told the nearest nurse. "We need an ortho consult, like yesterday." The nurse scurried to the phone, as Dr. Williamson began getting the story of what had happened.

Halfway through the history and physical exam, Dr. Sampson, the orthopedic surgeon on call, hit the double doors like a hammer and entered the trauma bay. "I hear we have a good one—" Suddenly, his eyes became dinner plates. "Son, can you feel that right foot of yours?"

"Holy shit, are you kidding me? This hurts so bad!"

"Yes, but your toes? Can you feel this?" Dr. Sampson pinched the toes of the right foot, which were all pointing in the wrong direction."

"Not really."

"I didn't think so, and they are already getting cold. This is going to be the worst pain of your life." That was it. That was the warning. I can't blame Dr. Sampson; if the nerves and blood supply were pinched, we were about to lose the foot. Dr. Sampson took the right foot in his meaty hands, pulled the foot laterally with his left hand, braced the patient's leg with his right, and snapped the foot back into alignment. The young man let out a blood-curdling scream, just about hit the ceiling, and let off a stream of epithets. "Alright, our open dislocation is now probably just an open fracture, and that is good. I will call the OR and get a room and my fracture kits ready. Send him down as soon as possible. There is probably dirt in that ankle." Dr. Sampson was out the trauma bay doors almost as fast as he had entered them.

"I think we could probably give him some morphine for pain. Start the IV for surgery, but give the first dose IM." Dr. Williamson, realizing there was probably not much more information he could glean from this screaming young man, and having assessed that there were no other injuries, signed off on his orders, and headed out of the trauma bay, "And get him down to surgery as soon as possible, please."

I could not believe what I had just seen and heard. I had seen dislocations relocated—at least half a dozen shoulders by this point—but had never seen an open dislocation relocated, and had never seen a joint relocation without sedation or anesthesia. Despite the fact that the foot had needed to be snapped back into place stat, it had still been terrible to watch someone go through it. Luckily, my day was almost over. Unfortunately, that screaming teenager haunted my dreams that night.

As my ED/trauma rotation drew to a close, I thought I had seen it all. Drug seekers, mad moms with children in no distress, foreign objects inserted where they didn't belong, car wrecks, and codes. I had even watched as Ndamukong Suh was drafted second overall in the NFL draft. My last shift at Creighton brought one more surprise. I was scheduled from 7 a.m. to 7 p.m. and since we were not on trauma coverage (it was a Friday), I figured there would not be anything all that noteworthy. I was wrong. At 5 p.m. we got our first drunk. The area surrounding Creighton is, to put it gently, low income. There are some nicer neighborhoods to the northwest in the Dundee area, but Creighton sits at the edge of "North O" and some of the poorest people, the Sudanese refugees, live nearby. Our refugee patient was quickly escorted to room 10, right behind me, as I wrapped up my rotation. The young man paced about the room, but did not come to the desk to hit on students, male or otherwise, so we didn't really worry about him. (All the cabinets in that room were locked since that was where we stored the suture kits, complete with needles.) I had almost forgotten about him when I heard the hissing sound of a stream of water hitting a flat surface. Our patient had apparently been looking for the restroom, and was now urinating on the wall, right over an electrical outlet. "Holy shit, he's pissing on the outlet!" I jumped up, was quickly met by a burly EMT, who then passed me at the door, and almost tackled the guy. The two of them fell against the wall, the EMT taking the brunt of the force, and slid to the floor. The drunken Sudanese gentleman, sans trousers, sat confused on top of an EMT who looked like a linebacker. A nurse arrived and we managed to hoist the patient off the EMT and get his britches up. As the EMT and I tried to convey the severity of the situation to the patient, the nurse called the police for a stat pick up. Our drunk was sober enough, thank you. Please come get him.

After housecleaning and maintenance left (they had to make sure there was no risk of a short in the outlet), my last day calmed down and ended without fanfare. Dr. Williamson was off that day, but I was able to say goodbye to Allison, the EMTs, and many of the nurses who had helped me survive my last (and most exciting) rotation. I certainly had no regrets about requesting CUMC and an extra two weeks by adding an elective. It was a high note to end on, but I was thankful my site coordinator had made it my last, not only because I enjoyed it, but had it been my first, as a naïve inexperienced PA student, I may have perished halfway through. The final drive back down to Lincoln was bittersweet as I left my most exciting rotation behind, but the excitement of my final tests and, barring any disaster on those, my approaching graduation certainly helped to soften the sadness.

Closing

"In medicine we are playing chess against God, and we are down a Bishop and all our pawns. You can extend the game; but you can never win." The first death on this clinical year was due to a Corn Nut lodged in a diverticulum. A Corn Nut killed my patient. The second death was due to colon cancer, regardless of how you consider her case. Prior to PA school the only cancer death I'd had any connection to was that of the grandmother I never met who was taken by ovarian cancer that had spread to her liver, lungs, and brain. Then during my clinical year I lost as many, if not more, patients to cancer as all other causes of death combined. I did not know it then, at the end of my clinical training, but years later I would watch my aunt successfully defeat breast cancer, survive past five years, then die of esophageal cancer. The board laid out, her oncologist moving the pieces around evading checkmate once, but still losing sooner than expected. My aunt, the grandmother I never met—their deaths would lead me to worry about the lone surviving female of that family: my mother. The woman who after one possibly bothersome annual exam would have not only her uterus but both ovaries removed based on family history and the fear of an early death.

I did not know it at the end of my clinical year, but my everyday life outside of work would forever be affected. Thanks to my pediatric rotation I would automatically screen every baby I held for a white pupil possibly revealing retinoblastoma, a cancer than can kill or blind if not treated quickly. Every time I'd get knee pain I would remember the Mormon missionary and how young he was when he presented with his football tumor—younger than me by a decade. I would see my children eating snacks they could choke on. I would see them riding bikes wearing helmets that may save their lives, but I'd think about how nothing could save them if the driver was going fast enough at the collision. I would worry about my own father on lipid-lowering drugs and antihypertensives and not be able to stop the fear that his heart attack was coming. I would try to trim every molecule of fat off my steak, knowing that with my paternal family history I should not even be eating steak or I too will have triple bypass surgery like my uncle and grandmother before me.

I have experienced death from every possible angle and cannot return to an existence where death is inevitable but distant. It has become my daily opponent. I cannot help but reflect on Thomas Gray's idea that ignorance is bliss, that if I did not know of death I would be happier. I try to remember Francis's chart; he smoked and drank, but not more so than others I have met. Was this the cause of his cancer? I do neither, yet know that cancer is sly when it comes for you. Growing out of a few cells whose reproduction has gone awry. There is no going back now.

I did indeed pass those final tests and graduated from physician assistant school a few weeks later. I passed the certification test on the first try and was soon off to Kansas City (Overland Park, in all actuality) for my first full-time job as a real physician assistant. My first job was in surgery, and I owe the scrub nurses in York, Nebraska, many thanks. Through their conditioning I had learned to hit the red line outside the surgical suites as if it were a brick wall, while I checked that my surgical cap and shoe covers were in place. Much like Pavlov's dog, they had conditioned me for the world of surgery. Kansas City was not my first choice. Sadly, I received a call from one of my first choices early in the week before accepting the Kansas City position, to say their budget had been cut and they could no longer offer me a position, only to have the budget improve the day after accepting my KC job. I am a man of my word and could not imagine rescinding my acceptance, so off to Kansas I went. There are many details, personal issues, and problems that made me feel as though I had to take that job in Kansas City. I don't believe this is the place to discuss those, since my focus here was to tell the story of a young man, armed only with classroom instruction and books, who, through personal experiences, becomes a true medical professional. I would like to write the next chapter of my journey: fresh-faced new graduate going into the world of medicine. If you are holding this book, yearning for more, rest assured that I am likely working on the next installment. I thank you for your support and hope you enjoyed reading about my journey as much as I enjoyed sharing it.

About the Author
Sean Conroy

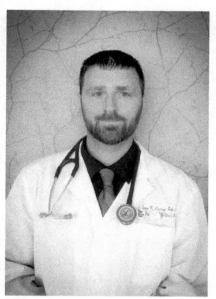

Sean Conroy was born and raised in McCook, Nebraska. He matriculated first from Chadron State College in Chadron, Nebraska with a bachelor's in biology (human biology option), then the University of Nebraska Medical Center in Omaha, Nebraska with a bachelor's in clinical laboratory science. He concluded his studies with a master's in physician assistant studies from Union College in Lincoln, Nebraska. He has practiced medicine in Kansas in primary care, including family practice and emergency medicine, since 2010.

CPSIA information can be obtained
at www.ICGtesting.com
Printed in the USA
LVHW092016051118
595973LV00009B/451/P

9 781941 799277